APPLIED RADIOGRAPHIC CALCULATIONS

APPLIED RADIOGRAPHIC CALCULATIONS

Cynthia A. Dennis, RT (R)

Program Director
Radiologic Technology Program
Louisiana State University
Shreveport, Louisiana

Ronald L. Eisenberg, MD, FACR

Chairman of Radiology
Highland General Hospital
Oakland, California
Clinical Professor of Radiology
University of California at San Francisco
San Francisco, California
and
University of California at Davis
Sacramento, California

W.B. SAUNDERS COMPANY
A Division of Harcourt Brace & Company
Philadelphia   London   Toronto   Montreal   Sydney   Tokyo

W.B. SAUNDERS COMPANY
A Division of Harcourt Brace & Company

The Curtis Center
Independence Square West
Philadelphia, Pennsylvania 19106

Library of Congress Cataloging-in-Pulication Data

Dennis, Cynthia A.
    Applied radiographic calculations / Cynthia A. Dennis. Ronald L.
Eisenberg.—1st ed.
        p.   cm.
    ISBN 0-7216-6596-9
    I. Radiography, Medical—Mathematics.   I. Eisenberg, Ronald L.
II. Title.
RC78.D444   1993
616.07′57′0151—dc20   92-28280

Applied Radiographic Calculations

ISBN 0-7216-6596-9

Printed in the United States of America

Last digit is the print number: 9   8   7   6   5   4   3   2

PREFACE

Radiologic technology students as well as practicing technologists frequently must rely on their knowledge of mathematics to make the calculations required to produce high-quality images. To meet this need, this book is designed to serve as both a review of general mathematics and a handy reference to the basic formulas and calculations used by radiographers. It begins with a review of basic mathematical principles such as addition, subtraction, multiplication, and division of whole numbers, mixed numbers, fractions, and decimals. There is also a review of ratio and proportion, basic principles of algebra and geometry, exponents, scientific notation, and metric conversions. Extensive work sheets filled with practice problems permit the student to thoroughly master each portion of the material in a step-by-step fashion.

Following the review sections, there is an introduction to the concepts and formulas necessary to solve various practical problems involving radiographic technique. Areas discussed include mAs conversions, inverse square law, radiographic density and contrast, screens and grid ratios, grid conversions, geometric and magnification unsharpness, graphs, and conversions between conventional and Système International (SI) units of radiation dosimetry. There is also a section introducing the formulas used in radiation physics. As in the review section, a wealth of sample problems are offered to permit the student to feel confident in having mastered the material.

The final part of the book offers a series of practical scenarios that reflect the various types of mathematical problems faced by radiologic technologists in clinical practice. These scenarios also serve to prepare the student for the types of problems encountered in classes on physics and radiation exposure as well as those faced by graduates on their A.R.R.T. registry examinations.

We want to express our thanks to Toiee Murray for the many hours she spent in the arduous task of typing and retyping the manuscript and the equations. We gratefully appreciate the superb line drawings of Carl Arthur Krebs, Jr., and the excellent photography of Stan Carpenter and Sheryl Austin of the Louisiana State University School of Medicine in Shreveport. Thanks should also go to the 1990–1992 classes of student technologists at LSU for reviewing the accuracy of the text as well as for making certain that we had the correct answers to the numerous examples and practical problems. Finally, we acknowledge the unceasing encouragement and support of Lisa Biello, Editor-in-Chief of Health-Related Professions at W.B. Saunders Company.

CYNTHIA A. DENNIS, RT (R)
RONALD L. EISENBERG, MD

CONTENTS

BASIC MATHEMATICAL CONCEPTS

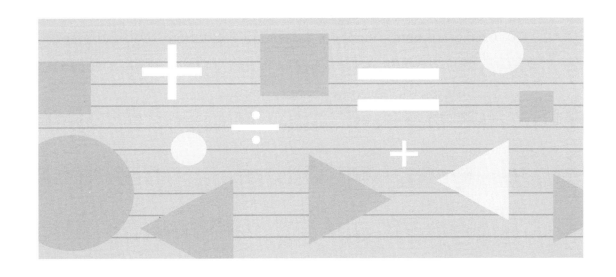

▼ OBJECTIVES SECTION ONE ▼

After completing this section, the student will be able to:

1. Perform addition, subtraction, multiplication, and division of fractions

2. Perform addition, subtraction, multiplication, and division of decimals

3. Change percent to decimal or fraction form

4. Increase or decrease numbers by a specified percentage

5. Set up ratios and proportions and prove that the proportions are true

6. Solve for one unknown using a proportion

7. Understand basic algebraic principles and solve for one unknown

8. Understand basic geometric principles and solve problems concerning circles, triangles, squares, and rectangles

9. Perform addition, subtraction, multiplication, and division using exponents

10. Change ordinary numbers to scientific notation form and vice versa

11. Perform metric and other conversions

Fractions

1. A **fraction** is a part of a whole number.

2. The top number is referred to as the **numerator**; the bottom number is referred to as the **denominator**.

3. A **proper** fraction has a value less than 1.

   Examples: $\frac{1}{5}$, $\frac{7}{8}$, $\frac{3}{7}$, $\frac{4}{9}$

4. An **improper** fraction has a value equal to or greater than 1.

   Examples: $\frac{1}{1}$, $\frac{8}{6}$, $\frac{10}{5}$, $\frac{9}{8}$

5. A **mixed number** contains a whole number and a fraction.

   Examples: $5\frac{1}{2}$, $4\frac{3}{4}$, $7\frac{1}{8}$, $3\frac{2}{3}$

6. A fraction is in its **lowest terms** when there is no number (divisor) that is common to both the numerator and denominator.

   Examples: $\frac{3}{5}$, $\frac{7}{9}$, $\frac{5}{6}$

7. A fraction can be reduced to its lowest terms by dividing the numerator and denominator by the largest number that is contained exactly in both.

   Example: $\frac{5}{10} = \frac{1}{2}$

   (5 goes into the numerator one time and into the denominator 2 times)

8. Any fraction can be changed to higher terms by multiplying both the numerator and the denominator by the same number.

   Example: $\frac{3}{5} = \frac{6}{10}$

   (3 multiplied by 2 equals 6; 5 multiplied by 2 equals 10)

9. Fractions can be added only if they have a **common denominator.** To find a common denominator, select the lowest number into which can be divided all the denominators to be added. For each fraction, multiply the numerator by the same number that must be multiplied by the denominator to equal the lowest common denominator.

   Example: $\frac{1}{4} + \frac{2}{3} + \frac{5}{6} = ?$

The lowest common denominator is 12

$$\frac{1}{4} = \frac{3}{12}$$
$$\frac{2}{3} = \frac{8}{12}$$
$$+ \frac{5}{6} = \frac{10}{12}$$
$$= \frac{21}{12} = 1\frac{9}{12} = 1\frac{3}{4}$$

* Note: Any answer resulting in an improper fraction should be changed to a mixed number. Any fraction in the answer should always be reduced to the lowest possible term.

10. Fractions can be subtracted only if they have a common denominator.

Example: $\frac{5}{8} - \frac{1}{3} = ?$

The lowest common denominator is 24

$$\frac{5}{8} = \frac{15}{24}$$
$$- \frac{1}{3} = \frac{8}{24}$$
$$= \frac{7}{24}$$

11. Fractions can be multiplied by multiplying the numerators and multiplying the denominators. If mixed numbers are to be multiplied, they must first be changed to improper fractions, and all fractions should be reduced to lowest possible terms prior to multiplying.

Example: $\frac{4}{5} \times \frac{3}{15} \times 1\frac{2}{8} =$
$\frac{4}{5} \times \frac{1}{5} \times \frac{10}{8} =$
$\frac{4}{5} \times \frac{1}{5} \times \frac{5}{4} = \frac{20}{100} = \frac{1}{5}$

12. Fractions can be divided by inverting the divisor and changing the sign to multiplication.

Example: $\frac{3}{8} \div \frac{2}{3} =$
$\frac{3}{8} \times \frac{3}{2} = \frac{9}{16}$

* Note: When multiplying or dividing you may cancel across signs.

Example: $\frac{4}{5} \times \frac{1}{5} \times \frac{5}{4} = \frac{1}{5}$

Example: $\frac{4}{5} \div 1\frac{3}{5} =$
$\frac{4}{5} \div \frac{8}{5} =$
$\frac{4}{5} \times \frac{5}{8} =$
$\frac{4}{8} = \frac{1}{2}$

▼ FRACTIONS WORK SHEET ▼

Perform each mathematical function indicated, reduce each answer to the lowest possible terms, and change any improper fraction to a mixed number.

1. $\frac{1}{8} \div \frac{4}{7} =$

2. $\frac{7}{9} - \frac{7}{18} =$

3. $\frac{1}{6} \div \frac{2}{3} =$

4. $1\frac{3}{8} - \frac{2}{3} =$

5. $2\frac{3}{4} \div 2\frac{1}{9} =$

6. $67\frac{1}{8} \times \frac{1}{4} =$

7. $\frac{8}{9} \div 1\frac{3}{5} =$

8. $7\frac{1}{3} - 6\frac{2}{3} =$

9. $122\frac{1}{3} \times \frac{1}{4} =$

10. $1\frac{3}{5} \div 2\frac{1}{9} =$

11. $3\frac{1}{17} - 1\frac{7}{34} =$

12. $\frac{6}{7} \times \frac{2}{9} \times \frac{14}{15} =$

13. $\frac{7}{16} + \frac{3}{4} + \frac{1}{8} =$

14. $\frac{3}{7} \times \frac{4}{5} \times \frac{1}{8} =$

15. $123\frac{4}{5} - 87\frac{3}{4} =$

16. $\frac{1}{4} + \frac{2}{5} + \frac{3}{8} =$

17. $2\frac{3}{8} \times 6\frac{2}{3} \times 3\frac{1}{2} =$

18. Divide $\frac{9}{15}$ by $\frac{3}{5} =$

19. $18\frac{3}{4} + \frac{6}{32} + 1\frac{5}{8} =$

20. $(\frac{3}{7} + \frac{2}{5}) \times (\frac{7}{9} \div \frac{2}{3}) =$

21. $\frac{8}{9} + \frac{7}{36} + 3\frac{1}{3} =$

22. $(\frac{1}{4} + \frac{7}{16}) - (\frac{3}{8} + \frac{4}{32}) =$

23. $1\frac{1}{5} + 2\frac{2}{3} + 3\frac{1}{6} =$

24. Multiply $\frac{4}{5}$ by $\frac{7}{9}$; then divide by $\frac{2}{3} =$

25. Divide $4\frac{2}{5}$ by $\frac{2}{3}$; then multiply by $3\frac{7}{8} =$

Decimals

1. A **decimal** is a fraction whose denominator is 10, 100, 1000, or any other multiple of 10.

2. The value of a decimal is determined by the place it holds to the right of the decimal point.

   Example: $0.5 = \frac{5}{10}$; $0.05 = \frac{5}{100}$; $0.005 = \frac{5}{1000}$

3. A decimal is read or named according to the place to the right of the decimal point (one number is tenths, two is hundredths, etc.).

   Examples: 0.624 is read as 624 thousandths
   0.0025 is read as 25 ten-thousandths

4. A decimal point serves to separate whole numbers from the decimal and is read using the whole number with the word "and" preceding the decimal.

   Examples: 6.0407 is read as six and four hundred and seven ten-thousandths
   300.006 is read as 300 and six thousandths

5. When adding or subtracting decimals, all decimal points must be placed in a vertical line.

   Example: $2.7 + 2.07 + 2.007 =$

$$
\begin{array}{r}
2.7 \\
2.07 \\
+\ 2.007 \\
\hline
6.777
\end{array}
$$

   Example: $8.97 - 6.3708 =$

$$
\begin{array}{r}
8.97 \\
-\ 6.3708 \\
\hline
2.5992
\end{array}
$$

6. When multiplying decimals, beginning from the right, count off as many decimal places in the product as there are in the multiplicand and multiplier combined.

Example: 2.968 × 4.05

$$\begin{array}{r} 2.968 \quad \text{(three decimal places)} \\ \times\ 4.05 \quad \text{(two decimal places)} \\ \hline 12.02040 \quad \text{(five decimal places)} \end{array}$$

7. When dividing by a decimal, move the decimal to the end of the divisor, move the decimal the same number of places to the right in the dividend, and place the decimal in the quotient directly above the one in the dividend.

Example: 48 ÷ 6.4

$$\begin{array}{r} 7.5 \\ 6.4\overline{)48.0} \\ 44\ 8 \\ \hline 3\ 20 \\ 3\ 20 \\ \hline 0 \end{array}$$

Example: 805 ÷ .46

$$\begin{array}{r} 17\ 50. \\ .46\overline{)805.00.} \end{array}$$

8. When changing fractions to decimals, divide the numerator by the denominator.

Example: ¾ = 0.75

9. When changing decimals to fractions, the numbers in the decimal become the numerator and are placed over the denominator, which is indicated by the number of decimal places.

Example: 0.0955 = 955/10000 = 191/2000

▼ DECIMALS WORK SHEET ▼

Change fractions to decimals.

1. $^8/_{10}$ =

2. $^{30}/_{10000}$ =

3. $^{95}/_{1000}$ =

4. $^{195}/_{100}$ =

Change decimals to fractions and then reduce them to lowest possible terms.

5. 0.03 =

6. 0.220 =

7. 0.0205 =

8. 0.00005 =

Add the following values:

9. $0.03 + 3.2 + 0.603 + 30.675 =$

10. $1.065 + 0.20 + 4.00045 + 28.2 =$

11. $23.1 + 31.03 + 2.675 + 0.926 =$

12. $3080.623 + 8.79 + 16.003 + 1000.0803 =$

Subtract the following values:

13. $4.635 - 2.946 =$

14. $231 - 0.9876 =$

15. $12.8942 - 0.3253 =$

16. $13 - 0.09406 =$

Multiply the following values:

17. 23 × 1.634 =

18. 235 × 0.302 =

19. 1.7 × 1.63 =

20. 1.302 × 0.72 =

Divide the following values. Carry out to three decimal places and drop the remainder.

21. 383 ÷ 0.023 =

22. 1.792 ÷ 0.382 =

23. 0.2468 ÷ 0.0320 =

24. 32.6 ÷ 0.03 =

25. 6.020 ÷ 0.0456 =

Percentages

1. A **percentage** is a special type of fraction in which the denominator is always 100.

2. The word *percent* literally means "per one hundred" and is indicated by the symbol %.

3. When performing mathematical computations, percentages are first changed to either decimal or fractional form.

Example: What is 33% of 300?

$$33\% = 0.33 = {}^{33}\!/_{100}$$

$$300 \times 0.33 = 99$$

or

$$300 \times {}^{33}\!/_{100} = 99$$

* Note: Radiographers must be familiar with the use of percentages, since most technical changes are in the form of a percentage of increase or decrease of the original factors.

4. To **increase** a number by a percentage you must add the percentage of increase to the original figure (100% **plus** the percentage of increase times the original amount).

Example: Increase 500 by 20%

$$500 \times 120\% \text{ or } 500 \times 1.2 = 600$$

5. To **decrease** a number by a percentage you must subtract the percentage of decrease from 100% and then multiply this figure by the original amount (100% **minus** the percentage of decrease times the original amount).

Example: Decrease 80 by 20%

$$100\% - 20\% = 80\%$$
$$80 \times 80\% \text{ or } 80 \times 0.8 = 64$$

▼ PERCENTAGES WORK SHEET ▼

Change the following percentages to decimal and fraction form.

	Decimal	**Fraction**
1. 57% =		=
2. 33% =		=
3. 120% =		=
4. 510% =		=

Increase the following numbers by the specified percentage.

5. Increase 240 by 30%.

6. Increase 30 by 20%.

7. Increase 380 by 70%.

8. Increase 200 by 50%.

9. Increase 100 by 200%.

10. Increase 50 by 350%.

Decrease the following numbers by the specified percentage.

11. Decrease 360 by 25%.

12. Decrease 245 by 45%.

13. Decrease 100 by 50%.

14. Decrease 680 by 95%.

15. Decrease 175 by 66%.

16. Decrease 33 by 33%.

Solve the following problems.

17. What is 30% of 500?

18. What is 200% of 200?

19. What is 75% of 350?

20. What is 60% of 680?

21. What is 20% of 40?

22. What is 80% of 400?

23. What is 150% of 300?

24. What is 250% of 50?

Ratios and Proportions

1. A **ratio** expresses the relation of two numbers by division and may be expressed in any of three ways:

   ⅔;   2 ÷ 3;   2 : 3

   (The signs /, ÷, and : are used to indicate division.)

2. A **proportion** is the expression of two equivalent ratios.

   Example: 6 : 10 :: 12 : 20

   This is read as "6 is to 10 as 12 is to 20" and could be written as ⁶/₁₀ = ¹²/₂₀.

3. The outside terms of a proportion are called **extremes,** and the inside terms are **means.**

   Example: 6 : 10 :: 12 : 20

   The extremes (first and fourth terms) are 6 and 20. The means (second and third terms) are 12 and 10.

4. In any proportion, one extreme is equal to the product of the means divided by the other extreme, and one mean is equal to the product of the extremes divided by the other mean.

$$\text{One extreme} = \frac{\text{Product of the means}}{\text{The other extreme}}$$

and

$$\text{One mean} = \frac{\text{Product of the extremes}}{\text{The other mean}}$$

Example: 6 : 10 :: 12 : 20

$$6 = \frac{10 \times 12}{20} = 6$$

$$20 = \frac{10 \times 12}{6} = 20$$

$$10 = \frac{6 \times 20}{12} = 10$$

$$12 = \frac{6 \times 20}{10} = 12$$

5. In any proportion, the product of the extremes is equal to the product of the means.

   Example: 6 : 10 :: 12 : 20

   $$6 \times 20 = 10 \times 12$$
   $$120 = 120$$

6. To solve a problem using a proportion:

   a. Let the first term of the proportion be x (the unknown).

   b. Let the second term be given a number that denotes the same kind of quantity as the required answer.

   c. To place the two remaining terms, determine whether x will be more or less than the second term.

      (1) If the answer is to be less, place the lesser of the two remaining numbers in the third place

      (2) If the answer is to be more, place the greater of the two remaining numbers in the third place

   * Note: Always place like terms over like terms.

   Example: If 1 inch (in) = 2.54 centimeters (cm), how many inches would equal 76.2 cm?

   x in : 1 in :: 76.2 cm : 2.54 cm

   Multiplying the means and extremes:

   $$(x)(2.54) = (1)(76.2)$$
   $$x = \frac{76.2}{2.54}$$
   $$x = 30 \text{ in}$$

   * Note: A radiographer may use these rules of proportion to determine a new mAs to use when changing the distance of the x-ray tube from the film. This is discussed at length in Section 2 (page 65).

▼ RATIOS AND PROPORTIONS WORK SHEET ▼

Write each of the following relations in the form of a proportion and prove that the proportion is true. Then multiply the means and the extremes to show that the proportion is correct.

1. 280 is to 560 as 1 is to 2.

2. 3 has the same relation to 36 as 12 has to 144.

3. 15 relates to 300 as 10 relates to 200.

4. ⅛ is to ¹⁄₃₂ as ¼ is to ¹⁄₁₆.

5. 0.33 relates to 99 as 0.22 is to 66.

Solve for x in the following proportions:

6. x is to 40 as 10 is to 400.

7. 30 is to x as 60 is to 90.

8. 240 is to 360 as x is to 1200.

9. 2 is to ⅛ as ¼ is to x.

10. x is to ⅓ as ¾ is to ½.

Algebraic Principles

1. **Algebra** provides a method of finding an unknown quantity that has a specific relation to one or more known quantities.

2. Algebraic operations are indicated by the same symbols used in arithmetic: $+$, $-$, $\times$, $\div$, $=$.

3. When solving any equation, you must keep the equation balanced by performing the same operation to both sides of the equation.

   Example: $4x - 8 = 12$
   $4x - 8 + 8 = 12 + 8$ (add 8 to both sides)
   $4x = 20$ (divide both sides by 4)
   $x = 5$

4. When solving equations, the unknown must be isolated by performing the inverse operations in a correct sequence. In the previous example, note that the first step was to isolate the unknown portion of the equation ($4x$) and the second step was to isolate the unknown (x). In both steps, the equation was kept balanced by performing the same operation on both sides of the equation, and in each case an inverse operation was required to isolate the unknown.

5. A formula may be solved for any of its components by using algebraic principles.

   Example: $mAs = mA \times s$

   To solve for **mA**, both sides of the equation must be divided by s:

   $$\frac{mAs}{s} = \frac{mA \times s}{s}$$

   $$\frac{mAs}{s} = mA$$

   To solve for **s**, both sides of the equation must be divided by mA:

   $$\frac{mAs}{mA} = \frac{mA \times s}{mA}$$

   $$\frac{mAs}{mA} = s$$

* Note: Remember this procedure, because it will be used extensively for setting manual (non-phototimed) radiographic techniques.

* Note: This diagram may help you remember the procedure. Cover up the factor you wish to find and you will see what mathematical procedures must be performed.

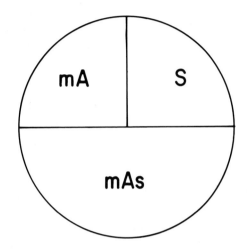

Example: To determine mA:
      1. Cover the mA portion of the circle.
      2. Divide mAs by s to get the mA.

Example: To determine mAs:
      1. Cover the mAs portion of the circle.
      2. Multiply mA by s to get the mAs.

▼ ALGEBRA WORK SHEET ▼

Solve for the specified unknown.

1. $a + b = cd$; $a =$

2. $a - b = cd$; $a =$

3. $\dfrac{a}{b} = cd$; $a =$

4. $\dfrac{a}{b} = \dfrac{c}{d}$; $c =$

5. $ab = cd$; $d =$

6. $ab = cd$; $b =$

7. $ab = cd$; $a =$

8. $ab = cd$; $c =$

9. $\dfrac{a}{b} = \dfrac{c}{d}$; $b =$

10. $\dfrac{a}{b} = \dfrac{c}{d}$; $d =$

11. $\text{mA}s = \text{mA} \times s$; $\text{mA} =$

12. $\text{mA}s = \text{mA} \times s$; $s =$

Solve for x.

13. $x + 12 = 64$

14. $x - 18 = 72$

15. $x + 122 = 186 - 46$

16. $x - 42 = 38 - 37$

17. $16x = 240$

18. $5x + 13 = 32$

19. $\frac{1}{2}x = 16 + 2$

20. $\frac{1}{2}x + \frac{1}{3} = \frac{1}{2}$

21. $1\frac{1}{2}x + \frac{2}{3} = \frac{4}{5} + \frac{1}{10}$

22. $\frac{4}{5}x = (3)(4)$

23. $-18 - 5x = 53$

24. $4x + 3x - 23 = 5x + x - 21$

25. $6x - 36 = 8x - 38$

Geometric Principles

I. Circles

A. A **circle** is defined as a curve all of whose points are an equal distance from the center.

B. The **circumference** (*C*) of a circle is the distance measured around the circle.

C. The **diameter** (*d*) of a circle is the distance measured across a circle. It also is equal to twice the radius.

D. The **radius** (*r*) of a circle is the distance measured from the center to any point on the circle. It is equal to ½ the diameter.

E. The Greek letter **pi** (π) designates the ratio of the circumference of a circle to its diameter. It is equal to 3.14159265+. For practical everyday use, π is rounded to 3⅐ (²²⁄₇) or 3.14.

F. The **area** of a circle = πr^2

Example: What is the area of a circle with a radius of 4 inches?

$$A = \pi r^2$$
$$A = 3.14 \times (4 \text{ in})^2$$
$$A = 3.14 \times 16 \text{ in}^2$$
$$A = 50.24 \text{ in}^2$$

* Note: The area of any figure is **always** expressed in square units.

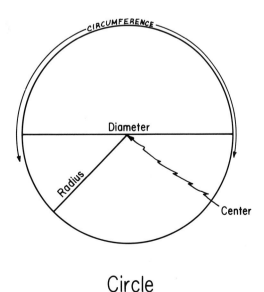

Circle

G. The **circumference** of a circle is equal to $2(\pi r)$ or πd or $\pi(2r)$.

Example: What is the circumference of a circle with a radius of 4 in?

$C = 2\pi r$
$C = 2(3.14 \times 4 \text{ in})$
$C = 2(12.56 \text{ in}) = 25.12 \text{ in}$

or

If radius = 4 in, diameter = 8 in

$C = \pi d$
$C = 3.14 \times 8 \text{ in}$
$C = 25.12 \text{ in}$

or

$C = \pi(2r)$
$C = 3.14 \times (2 \times 4 \text{ in})$
$C = 3.14 \times 8 \text{ in}$
$C = 25.12 \text{ in}$

▼ CIRCLES WORK SHEET ▼

1. What is the radius of a circle with a diameter of 6 in?

2. What is the radius of a circle with a diameter of ½ in?

3. What is the diameter of a circle with a radius of 1 in?

4. What is the diameter of a circle with a radius of 4 cm?

5. What is the circumference of a circle with a radius of 3 in?

6. What is the circumference of a circle with a diameter of 1 meter (m)?

7. What is the area of a circle with a radius of 2 cm?

8. What is the area of a circle with a radius of 1½ in?

9. What is the area of a circle with a diameter of 1 m?

10. What is the area of a circle with a diameter of ⅔ foot (ft)?

11. What is the diameter of a circle with a circumference of 31.4 in?

12. What is the radius of a circle with a circumference of 18.84 cm?

13. What is the area of a circle with a circumference of 9.42 ft?

14. What is the area of a circle with a circumference of 4.71 m?

15. What is the area of a circle with a circumference of 56.52 in?

II. Triangles

A. Triangles are classified by either **angles** or **sides**.

1. An **acute** triangle has three acute angles (less than 90°).

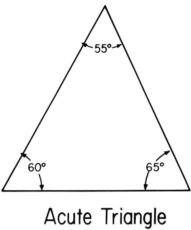

Acute Triangle

2. A **right** triangle contains one right angle (90°) and two acute angles.

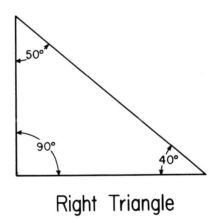

Right Triangle

3. An **obtuse** triangle has one obtuse angle (greater than 90°).

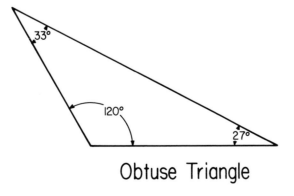

Obtuse Triangle

4. An **equilateral** triangle has three equal sides and three equal angles (60°).

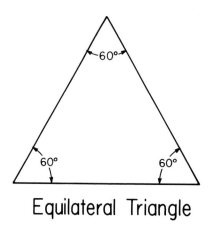

Equilateral Triangle

5. An **isosceles** triangle has two equal sides and two equal angles.

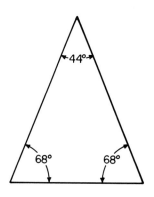

Isosceles Triangle

6. A **scalene** triangle has no equal sides or angles.

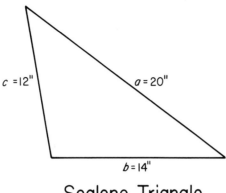

Scalene Triangle

B. The sum of the angles of **any** triangle is 180°.

Example: What is the third angle of a triangle whose other angles
are 60° and 80°?

$$\text{Angle 1} + \text{Angle 2} + \text{Angle 3} = 180°$$
$$60 + 80 + x = 180$$
$$140 + x = 180$$
$$x = 180 - 140$$
$$x = 40°$$

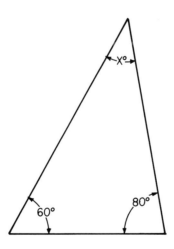

C. The **perimeter** (P) of any triangle is the sum of its three sides.

Example: What is the perimeter of a triangle whose sides are 10
cm, 14 cm, and 23 cm?

$$P = \text{Side 1} + \text{Side 2} + \text{Side 3}$$
$$P = 10 \text{ cm} + 14 \text{ cm} + 23 \text{ cm}$$
$$P = 47 \text{ cm}$$

D. The **Pythagorean theorem** can be used to determine the length of one side of a right triangle if the other two sides are known. The theorem states that the square of the long side opposite the right angle (the **hypotenuse**) is equal to the sum of the squares of the other two sides.

$$c^2 = a^2 + b^2$$

Example: What is the length of the hypotenuse of a right triangle whose other two sides are 6 and 8 in?

$c^2 = a^2 + b^2$
$c^2 = (6)^2 + (8)^2$
$c^2 = 36 + 64$
$c^2 = 100$
$c\ \ = 10$ in

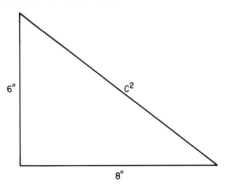

E. **Similar** triangles:

1. The corresponding angles are equal and the corresponding sides are proportional

$$x = X \qquad y = Y \qquad z = Z$$

2. A line drawn parallel to the base of any triangle will produce similar triangles

$$a = A \qquad b = B \qquad c = C$$

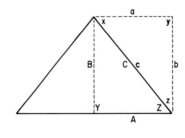

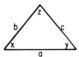

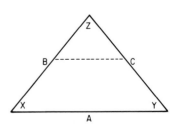

* Note: Of special interest to the radiographer are similar triangles. The proportional relationship of similar triangles must be understood if the radiographer is to understand the relationship of an image on a radiograph to the actual size of the object being projected. This is discussed at length in Section 2, page 111.

F. The **height** (altitude) of a triangle is a perpendicular line drawn
from any vertex (angle) to the opposite side (base).

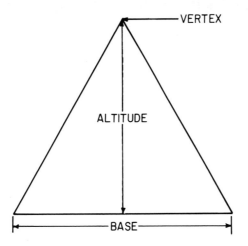

G. The **area** (A) of any triangle is equal to ½ the base (b) multiplied
by the height (h).

$$A = \frac{1}{2}bh$$

Example: What is the area of a triangle with a height of 7 in and a
base of 10 in?

$A = \frac{1}{2}bh$
$A = \frac{1}{2}(10 \times 7)$
$A = 35 \text{ in}^2$

* Note: Remember that the area is **always** expressed in square
units.

▼ TRIANGLES WORK SHEET ▼

1. What is the perimeter of a triangle with sides of 7 cm, 12 cm, and 23 cm?

2. What is the perimeter of a triangle with two sides of 10 cm and a base of 20 cm?

3. What is the length of the base of an isosceles triangle that has a perimeter of 60 in and one side of 15 in?

4. A triangle has a base of 18 in and another side of 12 in. If the perimeter is 38 in, how long is the third side?

5. What is the area of a triangle with a base of 10 cm and a height of 12 cm?

6. What is the area of a triangle with a height of 1 ft and a base of 18 in?

7. What is the area of a triangle with a height of 1½ ft and a base of 18 in?

8. What is the area of a triangle with a base of 14 cm and a height of 16 cm?

9. What is the length of the hypotenuse of a right triangle whose other two sides are 5 and 12 in?

10. What is the length of the hypotenuse of a right triangle whose other two sides are 6 and 8 in?

III. Rectangles

A. A **rectangle** is a four-sided figure whose opposite sides are equal.

B. The longer sides are referred to as the **length** (*l*) and the shorter sides are called the **width** (*w*).

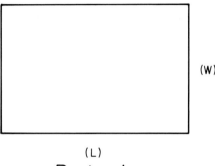

(W)

(L)

Rectangle

C. The **perimeter** (*P*) of a rectangle is determined by adding the measurements of the four sides (length plus width plus length plus width)

$$P = 2L + 2W$$

Example: What is the perimeter of a rectangle with a length of 6 ft and a width of 4.5 ft?

$P = 2L + 2W$
$P = (2 \times 6) + (2 \times 4.5)$
$P = 12 + 9$
$P = 21$ ft

D. The **area** (*A*) of a rectangle is determined by multiplying its length by its width.

$$A = L \times W$$

Example: What is the area of a rectangle with a length of 6 ft and a width of 4.5 ft?

$A = L \times W$
$A = 6 \times 4.5$
$A = 27$ ft^2

* Note: Remember that the area is **always** expressed in square units.

▼ RECTANGLES WORK SHEET ▼

1. What is the perimeter of a rectangle with a length of 9 in and a width of 4 in?

2. What is the area of a rectangle with a length of 3 ft and a width of 2 ft?

3. What is the width of a rectangle with a perimeter of 46 in and a length of 16 in?

4. What is the perimeter of a rectangle with a length of 1½ ft and a width of 6 in?

5. What is the width of a rectangle with a length of 17 in and a perimeter of 4 ft?

6. If a rectangle has an area of 12 in² and a width of 3 in, what is its length?

7. What is the perimeter of a rectangle with an area of 48 in² and a length of 8 in?

8. What is the area of a rectangle with a perimeter of 42 in and a width of 6 in?

9. What is the perimeter of a rectangle with an area of 864 in² and a length of 36 in?

10. What is the area of a rectangle with a perimeter of 6 ft and a length of 24 in?

IV. Squares

A. A **square** is a four-sided figure whose sides are equal in length (a rectangle with four equal sides).

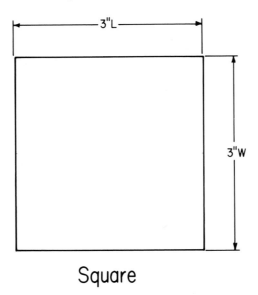

Square

B. The **perimeter** of a square is determined by adding the lengths of the four sides (S). More simply, the perimeter of a square equals 4 times the length of any side.

$$P = 4 \times S$$

Example: What is the perimeter of a square with sides measuring 5 ft?

$P = 4 \times S$
$P = 4 \times 5$
$P = 20$ ft

C. The **area** of a square is determined by multiplying the length of a side by itself, or (side)^2.

Example: What is the area of a square with sides measuring 5 ft?

$A = S^2$
$A = 5 \times 5$
$A = 25$ ft^2

* Note: Remember that area is **always** expressed in square units.

▼ SQUARES WORK SHEET ▼

1. What is the perimeter of a square with 1 side measuring 1½ ft?

2. If the area of a square is 169 in^2, what is the length of each side?

3. If each side of a square measures ⅞ ft, what is its perimeter?

4. If each side of a square measures 1⅔ ft, what is its area?

5. If a square has an area of 324 in^2 and a perimeter of 72 in, what is the length of each side?

Exponents

1. Exponents are a useful shorthand tool when it is necessary to repeatedly multiply a number by itself. The number 256 equals $2 \times 2 \times 2 \times 2 \times 2 \times 2 \times 2 \times 2$, or 2 times itself 8 times. In scientific problems this number can be expressed as 2^8. The repeated number (in this case 2) is called the **base**; the number of times the base is used as a multiplication factor (in this case 8) is termed the **exponent** or the **power** to which the base is raised. In this example 2^8 is read as "2 to the 8th power" or simply "2 to the 8th."

   Example: Write 100,000 as a power of 10.

   $$100,000 = 10 \times 10 \times 10 \times 10 \times 10 = 10^5$$

2. Certain powers are given special names. The second power is called the **square**; the third power is the **cube**.

   Example: What is the square of 12?

   $$12^2 = 12 \times 12 = 144$$

   Example: What is the cube of 9?

   $$9^3 = 9 \times 9 \times 9 = 729$$

3. To **multiply** two powers of the same number, simply **add** the exponents.

   Example: $2^3 \times 2^4 = 2^{3+4} = 2^7$

4. To **divide** two powers of the same number, simply **subtract** the exponents.

   Example: $3^8 \div 3^5 = 3^{8-5} = 3^3$

5. In division, if the power of the divisor is greater than the power of the dividend, the result is a **negative** power.

   Example: $4^3 \div 4^6 = 4^{3-6} = 4^{-3}$

   This is the same as $\dfrac{1}{4^3} = \dfrac{1}{4 \times 4 \times 4} = \dfrac{1}{64}$

6. If an exponent is placed outside parentheses, it is necessary to perform the operation inside the parentheses **before** raising the number to the indicated power.

   Example: $(4 \times 3)^2 = 12^2 = 144$

7. The **square root** of a number is that value which, when multiplied by itself, equals the number. The square root is usually represented by the radical sign: $\sqrt{}$.

   Example:

Number	Square Root
4	2
9	3
16	4
25	5
100	10

▼ EXPONENTS WORK SHEET ▼

Convert the following exponential expressions:

1. $9^2 =$

2. $40^2 =$

3. $72^2 =$

4. $30^2 =$

5. $36^2 =$

6. $44^2 =$

7. $48^2 =$

8. $60^2 =$

9. $4^3 =$

10. $8^4 =$

11. $2^7 =$

12. $3^9 =$

Solve the following problems.

13. $6^7 \div 6^4 =$

14. $8^5 \div 8^7 =$

15. $2^4 \div 2^6 =$

16. $3^3 \div 3^4 =$

17. $(6 \times 2)^2 =$

18. $(3 \times 2)^3 =$

19. $(6 \div 2)^4 =$

20. $(8 \div 4)^2 =$

21. $\sqrt{5184} =$

22. $\sqrt{900} =$

23. $\sqrt{1296} =$

24. $\sqrt{1600} =$

25. $\sqrt{1936} =$

26. $3^3 \times 3^2$

27. $4^4 \times 4^5$

28. $2^8 \times 2^{10}$

29. $8^2 \times 8^5$

30. $6^4 \times 6^7$

Scientific Notation

1. By using the exponential system of powers of 10, very large or very small numbers can be changed into a more convenient form.

2. **Large** numbers are written with the first significant digit placed to the left of the decimal point and any other significant numbers placed to the right of the decimal point. This number is then multiplied by a **positive** power of 10, which indicates the number of figures to the left of the decimal point when it is expressed in expanded form.

   Examples: 648,000,000,000 can be written as 6.48×10^{11}
   74,000,000 can be written as 7.4×10^7

3. **Small** numbers are written with the first significant number placed to the left of the decimal point and any other significant numbers placed to the right of the decimal point. This number is then multiplied by a **negative** power of 10, which indicates the number of figures to the right of the decimal point (including the first significant digit).

   Examples: 0.000000000000432 can be written as 4.32×10^{-13}
   0.000000400 can be written as 4×10^{-7}

4. To **multiply** numbers using scientific notation, first multiply the numbers before the powers of 10 and then add the exponents of the powers of 10.

   Example: Multiply 3.48×10^5 by 2.78×10^4

   Step 1: Multiply numbers before the powers of 10

   $3.48 \times 2.78 = 9.6744$

   Step 2: Add exponents of the powers of 10

   $5 + 4 = 9$

   Step 3: Multiply the product of Step 1 by the power of 10 in Step 2

   9.6744×10^9

   Example: $(7.689 \times 10^3) \times (2.34 \times 10^2) = 17.99226 \times 10^5$

5. To **divide** numbers using scientific notation, first divide the numbers before the powers of 10 and then subtract the exponents of the powers of 10.

   Example: Divide 9.99×10^8 by 3.33×10^4

   Step 1: Divide numbers before the powers of 10

   $$9.99 \div 3.33 = 3$$

   Step 2: Subtract exponents of the powers of 10

   $$8 - 4 = 4$$

   Step 3: Multiply the quotient in Step 1 by the power of 10 in Step 2

   $$3 \times 10^4$$

   Example: $(8.38 \times 10^9) \div (3.07 \times 10^{-6}) = 2.7206416 \times 10^{15}$

   * Note: When an exponent is moved from the denominator to the numerator, the sign is changed and the numbers added: $9 - (-6) = 9 + 6$.

6. To **add** or **subtract** numbers using scientific notation, the powers of 10 **must be the same**. The usual procedure is to convert the expression with the smaller exponent to one with the larger exponent. Digits do not have the same place value when written in decimal form. Therefore, **never** add or subtract the significant digit portion of the numbers if they do not have the same power of 10.

   Example 1: $(7.89 \times 10^4) + (6.92 \times 10^3)$

   $$
   \begin{array}{r}
   7.89 \times 10^4 \\
   +6.92 \times 10^3 \\
   \hline
   \end{array}
   \qquad
   \begin{array}{r}
   7.89 \times 10^4 \\
   +0.692 \times 10^4 \\
   \hline
   8.592 \times 10^4
   \end{array}
   $$

   Example 2: $(11.39 \times 10^{-5}) - (9.03 \times 10^{-7})$

   $$
   \begin{array}{r}
   11.39 \times 10^{-5} \\
   -9.03 \times 10^{-7} \\
   \hline
   \end{array}
   \qquad
   \begin{array}{r}
   11.39 \times 10^{-5} \\
   -0.0903 \times 10^{-5} \\
   \hline
   11.2997 \times 10^{-5}
   \end{array}
   $$

   or

   $$1.12997 \times 10^{-4}$$

* Note: The answer should always be written with the decimal point in the standard position for scientific notation.

* Note: In scientific notation the answer is rounded to the smallest place value to the right of the decimal point.

Example 1: 8.59×10^4

Example 2: 1.13×10^{-4}

▼ SCIENTIFIC NOTATION WORK SHEET ▼

I. Express the following numbers in scientific notation form.

1. 25

2. 450

3. 3,608

4. 84,792

5. 783,687

6. 1,387,720

7. 0.88

8. 0.009

9. 0.0807

10. 0.00000009820

II. Convert the following scientific notations to ordinary numbers.

1. 1.8×10^4

2. 1.96×10^5

3. 7.8×10^3

4. 4.3×10^6

5. 8.7×10^9

6. 9.6×10^{-1}

7. 8.9×10^{-7}

8. 4.6×10^{-5}

9. 3.85×10^{-3}

10. 7.6×10^{-2}

Metric and Other Conversions

Radiographers encounter measurements in both English and metric form and may be required to convert from one to the other. This can be done by setting up a simple ratio between known factors.

When making conversions from English to metric or vice versa it is helpful to know the following prefixes:

Prefix	Meaning	Abbreviation
Kilo	1000 X	k
Hecto	100 X	h
Deka	10 X	da

* Note: Any base unit (meter, liter, or gram) would have a value of 1 X.

Deci	$\frac{1}{10}$ X	d
Centi	$\frac{1}{100}$ X	c
Milli	$\frac{1}{1000}$ X	m
Micro	$\frac{1}{1,000,000}$ X	μ or mc
Nano	$\frac{1}{1,000,000,000}$ X	n

* Note: *Micro-* and *nano-* are used for very small measurements at the cellular, molecular, or atomic level. You will encounter these prefixes in your radiographic technique, radiation physics, protection, and biology classes.

It may help you remember the relationships between the prefixes by memorizing the order and remembering that they decrease by $\frac{1}{10}$ as you descend the list and increase by 10 as you ascend the list.

Examples:
centimeter (cm) = $\frac{1}{100}$ meter
kilovolt (kV) = 1000 volts
milliampere (mA) = $\frac{1}{1000}$ ampere
milliliter (ml) = $\frac{1}{1000}$ liter
milligram (mg) = $\frac{1}{1000}$ gram
millimeter (mm) = $\frac{1}{1000}$ meter
millirad (mrad) = $\frac{1}{1000}$ rad

Example: 100 kilovolts is equal to _____ volt(s)
100 × 1000 volts = 100,000 volts

Example: 100 milliamperes is equal to _____ ampere(s)
100 × $\frac{1}{1000}$ ampere = $\frac{1}{10}$ ampere

Example: 100 centimeters is equal to _____ meter(s)
           $100 \times 1/100$ meter = 1 m

Example: 5 meters is equal to _____ centimeters(s)
           $1/100$ m = 1 cm and 100 cm = 1 m
           5×100 cm = 500 cm

Several common conversions are listed below.

Units of Time

$$1 \text{ millisecond} = 1/1000 \ (0.001) \text{ second}$$
$$1 \text{ second} = 1/60 \text{ minute}$$
$$1 \text{ minute} = 1/60 \text{ hour}$$
$$1 \text{ hour} = 1/24 \text{ day}$$

Example: 45 seconds is equal to what part of a minute?

$$1 \text{ sec } = 1/60 \text{ min}$$
$$45 \text{ sec} = 45/60 = 3/4 \text{ min}$$

Units of Temperature

Centigrade temperature = $5/9$ (Fahrenheit temperature − 32)

Example: 94° F is equal to _____° C.

$$C = 5/9 \ (F - 32)$$
$$C = 5/9 \ (94 - 32)$$
$$C = 5/9 \ (62)$$
$$C = 34.4°$$

Fahrenheit = ($9/5$ Centigrade) + 32

Example: A temperature of 20° C is equal to _____° F.

$$F = 9/5 \ C + 32$$
$$F = 9/5 \ (20) + 32$$
$$F = 36 + 32$$
$$F = 68° C$$

* Note: You can use a proportion as follows:

$$\frac{212° \text{ F} - 32° \text{ F}}{100° \text{ C} - 0° \text{ C}} = \frac{180}{100} = 1.8$$

$$\text{F} - 32 = \text{C} \times 1.8 \quad \text{or} \quad \text{F} = (\text{C} \times 1.8) + 32$$

$$\text{C} = \frac{\text{F} - 32}{1.8}$$

Liquid Measures

30 milliliters (ml) = 1 ounce (oz)
16 ounces = 1 pint (pt)
2 pints = 1 quart (qt)
1000 milliliters = 1 liter (L)
1 liter = 1.0567 quarts
1 quart = 0.946 liter
4 quarts = 1 gallon (gal)

Example: How many milliliters are there in 1 pint?

1 pt = 16 oz
1 oz = 30 ml
1 pt = 16 × 30 = 480 ml

Linear Measures

1 inch = 2.54 centimeters or 25.4 millimeters
12 inches = 1 foot
3 feet = 1 yard
1 mile = 5280 feet

Example: How many centimeters are there in 40 inches?

2.54 cm = 1 inch
2.54 × 40 = 101.6 cm

Weight

16 ounces = 1 pound (lb)
1 pound = 2.2 kilograms (kg)

Example: A weight of 80 lb equals _____ kg.

1 lb = 2.2 kg
2.2 × 80 = 176 kg

Household Measures

* Note: Household measures should never be used to measure exact amounts of medication or chemicals because there is too much variation depending on whether one is measuring a liquid or dry material.

1 teaspoon = ⅛ fluid ounce or 1 dram
3 teaspoons = 1 tablespoon
1 tablespoon = ½ fluid ounce or 4 drams
16 tablespoons (liquid) = 1 cup
12 tablespoons (dry) = 1 cup
1 cup = 8 fluid ounces or ½ pint

Example: If 3 oz of liquid is to be measured using a tablespoon, how many tablespoons would be used?

1 tablespoon = ½ ounce
2 tablespoons = 1 ounce
2 × 3 = 6 tablespoons = 3 ounces

▼ METRIC AND OTHER CONVERSIONS WORK SHEET ▼

1. The length of a patient's humerus is 15 in. What would this measurement be in centimeters?

2. How many milliliters are needed to fill an 8-oz bottle?

3. How many centimeters are there in 72 in?

4. How many meters are there in 72 in?

5. How many ounces make a quart?

6. How many yards are in a mile?

7. A temperature of 42° C is equivalent to _____° F.

8. A temperature of 88° F is equivalent to _____° C.

9. How many centimeters are in a mile?

10. How many milliliters are in 4 L?

11. 40 msec is equal to _____ sec.

12. 180 msec is equal to _____ sec.

13. 5 msec is equal to _____ sec.

14. 500 msec is equal to _____ sec.

15. 0.035 sec is equal to _____ msec.

16. 0.001 sec is equal to _____ msec.

17. 0.3 sec is equal to _____ msec.

18. 0.1 sec is equal to _____ msec.

19. ⁶/₁₀ sec is equal to _____ msec.

20. ²/₅ sec is equal to _____ msec.

RADIOGRAPHIC CALCULATIONS

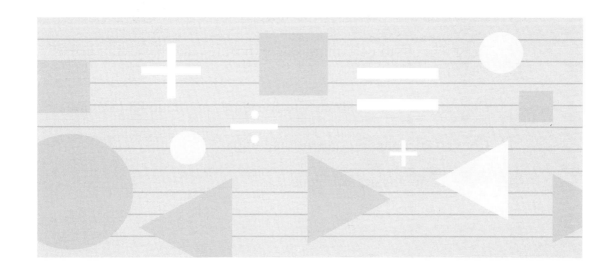

▼ OBJECTIVES SECTION TWO ▼

After completing this section, the student will be able to:

1. Solve problems for mA, time, and mAs

2. Use the inverse square law to solve for radiation intensity and dose

3. Use a variation of the inverse square law to solve for the new mAs needed when a source–image receptor distance is changed

4. Change the density of a radiograph using mAs

5. Change the scale of contrast on a radiograph using kVp

6. Change the density of a radiograph using kVp

7. Adjust radiographic techniques for various screen speed changes

8. Determine grid ratios

9. Adjust radiographic techniques for various grid ratio changes

10. Determine the amount of geometric unsharpness

11. Determine the percentage of magnification on a radiograph

12. Read a graph to determine safe exposures and basic film sensitometry

13. Convert conventional units to Système International (SI) units

14. Convert SI units to conventional units

15. Solve basic physics problems

mAs Conversions

When setting manual techniques for various radiographic procedures, two important factors are the **milliamperage** and **time** (in seconds). Milliamperage controls the amount of radiation; the time of exposure controls the period that a particular quantity or amount of radiation will be emitted from the x-ray tube. Together, the two control the density, or the degree of blackness, of the resulting radiograph.

Owing to differences in patients and equipment it is sometimes necessary to change either the milliamperage or the time of exposure without changing the desired density of the radiograph. This can be accomplished by keeping a constant mAs, which is equal to the milliamperage multiplied by the time of the exposure (mAs = mA × s).

By performing simple algebraic operations, the radiographer can easily calculate the mAs of any given exposure and then determine several combinations of mA and time that will produce similar radiographic exposures.

Example: A radiograph is produced using 300 mA for 0.035 sec. What is the mAs?

mAs = mA × s
mAs = 300 × 0.035
mAs = 10.5

Example: A radiograph is produced using 100 mA for 0.4 sec. What is the mAs?

100 × 0.4 = 40 mAs

What time of exposure could be used with 200 mA to produce 40 mAs?

mAs = mA × s

$$s = \frac{mAs}{mA}$$

$$s = \frac{40}{200}$$

s = ⅕ = 0.2 sec

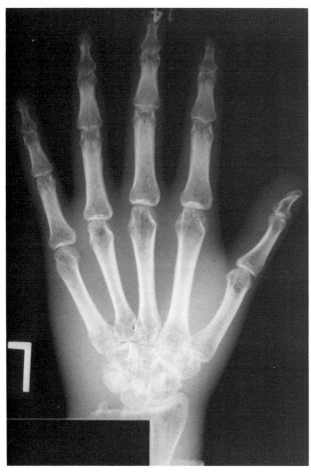

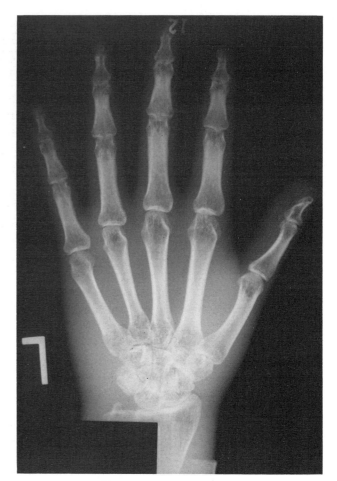

100 mA at 0.01 s (1 mAs)   50 mA at 0.019 s (0.95 mAs)

What mA could be used with ¹/₁₀ (0.1) sec to produce 40 mAs?

$$mAs = mA \times s$$

$$mA = \frac{mAs}{s}$$

$$mA = \frac{40}{0.1}$$

$$mA = 400$$

or

$$mA = 40 \div \frac{1}{10}$$
$$mA = 40 \times \frac{10}{1} = 400$$

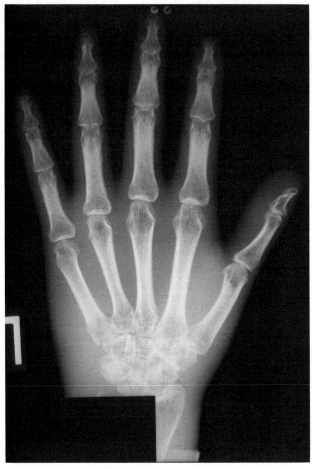

200 mA at 0.05 s (1 mAs)

* Note: Remembering this diagram might be helpful in remembering
the relationships of mA and time to mAs:

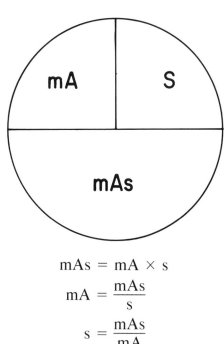

$$mAs = mA \times s$$

$$mA = \frac{mAs}{s}$$

$$s = \frac{mAs}{mA}$$

▼ mAs CONVERSIONS WORK SHEET ▼

A. Give the mAs value for the following mA and time combinations:

1. 400 mA $^1\!/_{120}$ sec   = 3.33

   $\dfrac{400}{1} \cdot \dfrac{1}{120}$

2. 600 mA $^1\!/_{30}$ sec   = 20 mas

3. 500 mA $^1\!/_5$ sec   = 100
   .2

4. 200 mA $^3\!/_{10}$ sec   = 60
   .3

5. 50 mA $^1\!/_{40}$ sec   = 1.25

6. 100 mA $^1\!/_{15}$ sec   = 6.66

7. 300 mA $^1\!/_{10}$ sec   = 30

8. 100 mA $^3\!/_{20}$ sec   = 15

9. 600 mA $^2\!/_5$ sec   = 240

10. 500 mA $^1\!/_{40}$ sec   = 125

B. For the following mA and time combinations state the appropriate mAs:

1. 300 mA   0.035 sec   = 10.5

2. 400 mA   0.025 sec   = 10

3. 600 mA   0.01 sec   = 6

4. 500 mA   0.4 sec   = 200

5. 100 mA   0.01 sec   = 1

6. 200 mA   0.02 sec   = 4

7. 300 mA   0.07 sec   = 21

8. 500 mA   0.35 sec   = 175

9. 50 mA   0.035 sec   = 1.75

10. 600 mA   0.25 sec   = 150

C. For the following mAs and time give the required milliamperes (mA):

$MA \cdot S = MAS$

$MA = \frac{MAS}{S}$

1. 6.66 mAs   0.067 sec   =   99.4

2.   30 mAs   0.1 sec   =   300

3.   75 mAs   3/20 sec   =   500

$\frac{75}{1} \div \frac{3}{20} = \frac{75}{1} \times \frac{20}{3}$

4.   15 mAs   0.025 sec   =   600

5.   40 mAs   1/10 sec   =   400

$\frac{40}{1} \div \frac{1}{10} = \frac{40}{1} \times \frac{10}{1} =$

6.   70 mAs   0.35 sec   =   24.5

7.   375 mAs   3/4 sec   =   500

8.   3.3 mAs   1/60 sec   =   198

$\frac{3.3}{1} \div \frac{1}{60} = \frac{3.3}{1} \times \frac{60}{1} =$

9.   120 mAs   0.4 sec   =   300

10.   7.5 mAs   3/10 sec   =   25

$7.5 \div \frac{3}{10} = \frac{2.5}{1} \times \frac{10}{3}$

D. For the following mAs and mA combinations give the appropriate time in both decimal and fraction form:

mA·S = mAS

$\frac{mAS}{mA}$ = S

1. 1.25 mAs   100 mA = .0125   = $\frac{1}{80}$ sec

2.   50 mAs   400 mA = .125   =   sec

3.   10 mAs   500 mA = .02   = $\frac{1}{50}$ sec

4.   40 mAs   600 mA = .066   =   sec

5. 0.5 mAs   50 mA = .01   = $\frac{1}{100}$ sec

6. 150 mAs   300 mA = .5   = $\frac{1}{2}$ sec

7.   5 mAs   400 mA = .0125   = $\frac{1}{80}$ sec

8.   60 mAs   400 mA = .15   = $\frac{3}{20}$ sec

9.   80 mAs   200 mA = .4   = $\frac{2}{5}$ sec

10. 300 mAs   400 mA = .75   = $\frac{3}{4}$ sec

Introduction to the Inverse Square Law

The **inverse square law** states that the intensity of radiation is inversely proportional to the square of the distance between the x-ray tube and the image receptor (film). Using this law, it is possible for radiographers to determine the dose of radiation at a new distance if the dose at the original distance is known. The following formula is used:

$$\frac{\text{New intensity}}{\text{Old intensity}} = \frac{\text{Old distance}^2}{\text{New distance}^2}$$

or

$$\frac{I_2}{I_1} = \frac{D_1^{\,2}}{D_2^{\,2}}$$

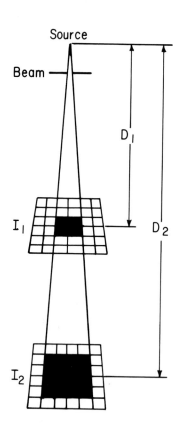

Example: If the radiation dose to a patient was 10 milliroentgens (mR) at a 40-in distance, what would the dose be if the distance were reduced to 30 in?

$$\frac{x}{10 \text{ mR}} = \frac{(40)^2}{(30)^2}$$

$$\frac{x}{10 \text{ mR}} = \frac{1600}{900}$$

$$\frac{x}{10 \text{ mR}} = \frac{16}{9}$$

$$9x = 160 \text{ mR}$$

$$x = 17.77 \text{ mR}$$

* Note: As the distance is decreased, the patient dose is increased.

Example: If the radiation dose to a patient is 10 mR at a distance of 40 in, what would the dose be at a distance of 60 in?

$$\frac{x}{10 \text{ mR}} = \frac{(40)^2}{(60)^2}$$

$$\frac{x}{10 \text{ mR}} = \frac{1600}{3600}$$

$$\frac{x}{10 \text{ mR}} = \frac{16}{36}$$

$$36x = 160 \text{ mR}$$

$$x = 4.44 \text{ mR}$$

* Note: As the distance is increased, the patient dose is decreased.

A variation of the inverse square law is used to establish the relation between mAs and the distance between the x-ray tube and image receptor (film), which is termed the focal-film distance (FFD), and the density produced on a radiograph. This permits the radiographer to determine what new mAs is needed if the distance is changed. The mAs (mA and time) varies **directly** with the square of the distance. The following formula is used:

$$\frac{\text{New mAs}}{\text{Old mAs}} = \frac{\text{New distance}^2}{\text{Old distance}^2}$$

or

$$\frac{mAs_2}{mAs_1} = \frac{D_2^2}{D_1^2}$$

Example: If 10 mAs was used to produce a satisfactory radiograph at a 40-in distance, what mAs would be required at a distance of 60 in?

$$\frac{x}{10 \text{ mAs}} = \frac{(60)^2}{(40)^2}$$

$$\frac{x}{10 \text{ mAs}} = \frac{3600}{1600}$$

$$\frac{x}{10 \text{ mAs}} = \frac{36}{16}$$

$$16x = 360 \text{ mAs}$$

$$x = 22.5 \text{ mAs}$$

* Note: As the distance is increased, the mAs must also be increased to maintain equal density.

Example: If a satisfactory radiograph was obtained using 10 mAs at a 40-in distance, what mAs would be required at a distance of 30 in?

$$\frac{x}{10 \text{ mAs}} = \frac{(30)^2}{(40)^2}$$

$$\frac{x}{10 \text{ mAs}} = \frac{900}{1600}$$

$$\frac{x}{10 \text{ mAs}} = \frac{9}{16}$$

$$16x = 90 \text{ mAs}$$

$$x = 5.6 \text{ mAs}$$

* Note: As the distance is decreased, the mAs must also be decreased to maintain equal density.

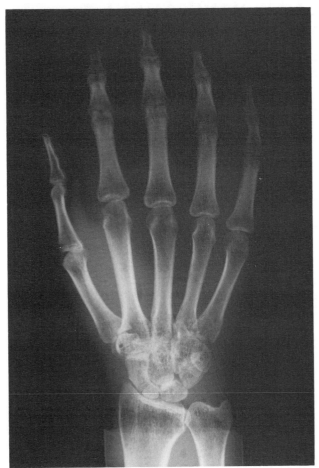

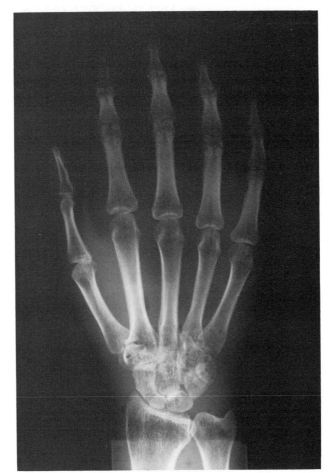

36 in SID at 1 mAs   48 in SID at 1.6 mAs

* Note: A shorter method of working the inverse square law, and one that does not involve such large numbers, is to simply divide the new distance by the old distance, square the result of this division, and then multiply by the old mAs.

Example: Using the same example as above,

$$\frac{30}{40} = \frac{3}{4}$$
$$\tfrac{3}{4} = 0.75$$

$$(\tfrac{3}{4})^2 = \tfrac{9}{16}$$
$$\tfrac{9}{16} \times 10 \text{ mAs} = 5.6 \text{ mAs}$$

or

$$(0.75)^2 = 0.5625$$
$$0.5625 \times 10 \text{ mAs} = 5.6 \text{ mAs}$$

▼ INVERSE SQUARE LAW WORK SHEET ▼

I. If the technique chart states that you should use a particular mAs for a procedure at a specified distance and you must change the distance, what new mAs would be required at the new distances listed in the problems below?

	Original			New	
	Distance (in)	mAs		Distance (in)	mAs
1.	40	400			
2.	44	240			
3.	36	150			
4.	30	75			
5.	48	90			
6.	60	320			
7.	72	480			
8.	30	3⅓			

Handwritten work:

1. $\frac{(60)^2}{(40)^2} = \frac{X}{400}$ $\frac{3600}{1600} = \frac{X}{400}$ 900
   $16X = 144000$

2. $\frac{(40)^2}{(44)^2} = \frac{X}{240}$ $\frac{1600}{1936} = \frac{X}{240}$ 198.
   $1936X$

3. $\frac{(30)^2}{(36)^2} = \frac{X}{150}$ $\frac{900}{1296} = \frac{X}{150}$ 104.16
   $1296X = 135000$

4. $\frac{(44)^2}{(30)^2} = \frac{X}{75}$ $\frac{1936}{900} = \frac{X}{75}$ 161.33

5. $\frac{(36)^2}{(48)^2} = \frac{X}{90}$ $\frac{1296}{2304} = \frac{X}{90}$ 50.625

6. $\frac{(72)^2}{(60)^2} = \frac{X}{320}$ $\frac{5184}{3600} = \frac{X}{320}$ 460.8

7. $\frac{(66)^2}{(72)^2} = \frac{X}{480}$ $\frac{4356}{5184} = \frac{X}{480}$ 403.33

8. $\frac{(36)^2}{(30)^2} = \frac{X}{3.33}$ $\frac{1296}{900} = \frac{X}{3.33} = 4.7$

9.   42   6.66 $\frac{(48)^2}{(42)^2} = \frac{x}{6.66}$ $\frac{2304}{1764} : \frac{x}{6.66} = 8.698$

10.   48   12⅔ $\frac{(44)^2}{(48)^2} = \frac{x}{12.66}$ $\frac{1936}{2304} = \frac{x}{12.66}$ 10.637

II. For the following problems, work out the new mAs required and give a new mA and time in fraction form that will give you the desired mAs. Remember that it is not always possible to get the exact mAs with the mA and time combinations available on your x-ray equipment. Choose an mA and time that are reasonable for your equipment. (Note that usually there will be more than one reasonable combination from which to select.)

	Original				New		
	Distance (in)	mA	Time (sec)	mAs	Distance (in)	mA	Time (sec)
1.	40	100	½		44		
2.	36	50	¼		30		
3.	44	600	0.035		60		
4.	30	300	0.02		36		
5.	48	1000	1/60		40		

III. For the following problems, work out the new mAs and give a new mA and time in decimal form that will give you the desired mAs. Remember that it is not always possible to get the exact mAs with the mA and time combinations available on your x-ray equipment. Choose an mA and time that are reasonable for your equipment.

	Original				New		
	Distance (in)	mA	Time (sec)	mAs	Distance (in)	mA	Time (sec)
1.	72	300	0.15		60		
2.	48	800	0.07		44		
3.	40	500	0.4		36		
4.	30	150	1/40 .025		48		
5.	44	25	3/4		72		

IV. For the following examples, determine the new radiation dose
the patient receives after a change in distance.

$\frac{I_1}{I_2} = \frac{(D_2)^2}{(D_1)^2}$

| | Original | | New | |
	Distance (in)	Radiation Dose (mR)	Distance (in)	Radiation Dose (mR)
1.	40	5	36	6.17 mR
		$\frac{5}{X} = \frac{1296}{1600}$		
2.	72	2½	60	
3.	48	8	72	
4.	36	25	40	
5.	30	50	44	
6.	60	10	72	
7.	66	7	60	
8.	50	4	40	
9.	50	4	60	
10.	50	4	30	

Introduction to Density Problems

Because of technologist error, equipment malfunction, or patient variation or pathology, it is occasionally necessary to change the density of a radiograph. Using a fixed-kilovoltage technique, the density can be changed by altering the mAs. This can be accomplished by changing either the mA or the time of exposure.

The request for a change in density is usually expressed as a percentage increase or decrease. By assessing the characteristics of the equipment and the clinical condition of the patient, the radiographer must determine whether to change the mA or the time to achieve the desired density. For example, if the density must be increased for a patient who is unable to hold his breath, it would be better to increase the mA and use the shortest time possible. If the patient is totally cooperative and motion is not a factor, it may be wiser to change the time to increase density, since changing mA stations may not always reflect the expected change, owing to improper calibration.

Example: Increase the density of a radiograph by 40%. The original technique was 100 mAs at 400 mA for 0.25 sec.

Step 1: Determine new mAs

100 mAs × 40% = 100 mAs × 0.4 = 40
100 mAs + 40 mAs = 140 mAs

or

100 mAs × 140% = 140 mAs

To determine what new mA and/or time would be required to achieve the mAs of 140, use the mAs formulas given in the mAs conversion section on pages 57 to 59. Depending on the type of equipment used, several possible combinations are these:

400 mA for 0.35 sec
200 mA for 0.7 ($^7/_{10}$) sec
100 mA for 1.4 sec

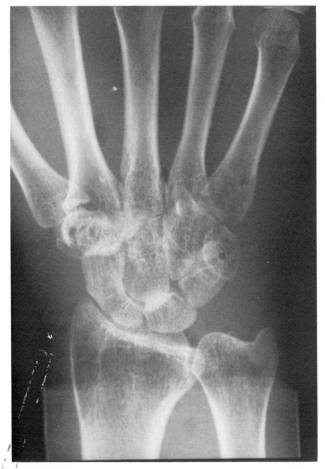

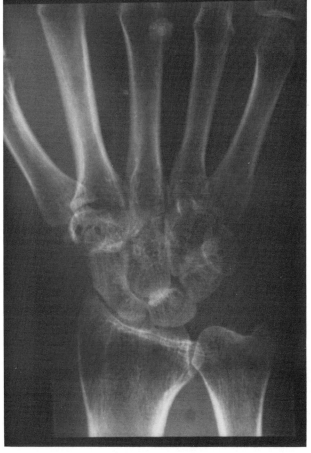

55 kVp at 1 mAs   55 kVp at 2 mAs (100% increase)

Example: Decrease the density of a radiograph by 30%. The original
technique was 85 kVp (kilovoltage peak) at 300 mA for $\frac{3}{5}$
(0.6) sec.

Step 1: Determine initial mAs

$$300 \times \frac{3}{5} = 180 \text{ mAs}$$

or

$$300 \times 0.6 = 180 \text{ mAs}$$

Step 2: Determine new mAs

$$180 \times 30\% = 180 \times 0.3 = 54$$
$$180 - 54 = 126 \text{ mAs}$$

or

$$180 \times 70\% = 126 \text{ mAs}$$

Step 3: Determine what mA station and what length of exposure would produce the desired mAs of 126.

As in this example, it is not always possible to find an mA and time that produce the exact mAs. It is often necessary to choose an mA and time that give the closest possible mAs to that desired.

Possible combinations for 126 mAs are:

300 mA for 0.4 sec = 120 mAs
600 mA for 0.2 sec = 120 mAs
800 mA for 0.15 sec = 120 mAs

* Note: A loss of 6 mAs at the 126-mAs level will not be perceptible on the radiograph. It is important to remember that **a change in mAs of at least 30% is necessary to produce an appreciable change in density** on a radiograph.

Example: A radiograph needs to be repeated using 60% of the original density. The original technique used was 85 kVp at 200 mA for 4/5 (0.8) sec.

Step 1: Determine initial mAs

200 × 4/5 = 160 mAs

Step 2: Determine new mAs

160 × 60% = 96 mAs

Possible combinations of mA and time to achieve 96 mAs are these:

200 mA for 0.5 sec = 100 mAs
400 mA for 0.25 sec = 100 mAs
600 mA for 0.15 sec = 90 mAs
800 mA for 0.125 sec = 100 mAs
1000 mA for 0.1 sec = 100 mAs

* Note: These slight changes in desired mAs would **not** cause a perceptible change in density.

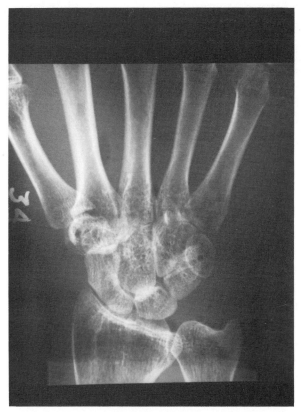

55 kVp at 1 mAs

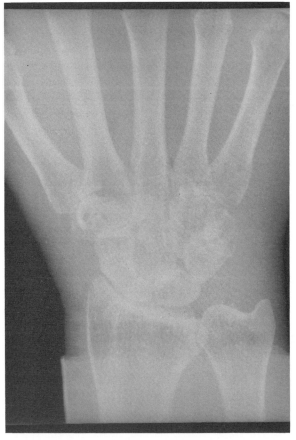

55 kVp at 0.5 mAs (50% decrease)

Example: A technique of 90 kVp at 600 mA for 0.03 sec produced a radiograph that needed a 50% increase in density to be diagnostic. What new mAs would be needed to achieve this 50% increase in density?

Step 1: Determine initial mAs

$600 \times 0.03 = 18$ mAs

Step 2: Determine new mAs

$18 \times 150\% = 27$ mAs

Possible combinations of mA and time to achieve 27 mAs are these:

400 mA for 0.06 sec = 24 mAs
500 mA for 0.05 sec = 25 mAs
600 mA for 0.04 sec = 24 mAs
800 mA for 0.03 sec = 24 mAs

Example: A radiograph obtained using 80 kVp at 800 mA for 0.007 sec was too light and required a 100% increase in density to achieve a diagnostic level. What new mAs must be used and what possible combinations of mA and time could be employed?

Step 1: Determine initial mAs

$800 \times 0.007 = 5.6$ mAs

Step 2: Determine new mAs

$5.6 \times 200\% = 11.2$ mAs

Possible combinations of mA and time to achieve 11.2 mAs are these:

400 mA for 0.025 sec = 10 mAs
400 mA for 0.03 sec   = 12 mAs
600 mA for 0.02 sec   = 12 mAs
800 mA for 0.015 sec = 12 mAs

Example: Using the initial technique in the previous example, determine the new mA and time required to increase the density by 200%.

Step 1: Determine the initial mAs

$800 \times 0.007 = 5.6$ mAs

Step 2: Determine the new mAs

$5.6 \times 300\% = 16.8$ mAs

Possible combinations of mA and time to achieve 16.8 mAs are these:

600 mA for 0.03 sec = 18 mAs
800 mA for 0.02 sec = 16 mAs

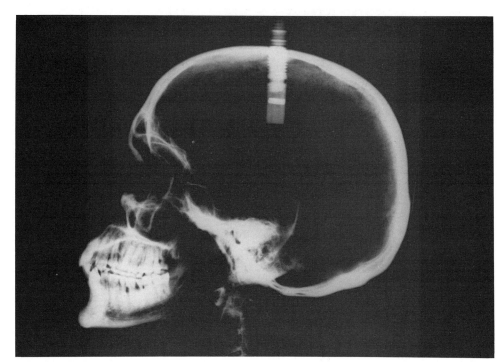

Original

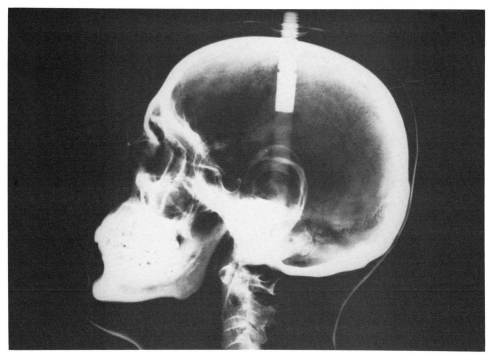

60% decrease in density

▼ DENSITY PROBLEMS WORK SHEET ▼

1. The density of a radiograph must be reduced by 40%. The original technique was 90 kVp at 60 mAs. What new mAs must be used?

2. A radiograph needs to be repeated using 75% of the original density. The original technique used was 75 kVp at 300 mA for ⅕ sec. What new mAs would be required?

3. A radiograph was obtained using 70 kVp at 600 mA for 0.025 sec. The radiograph was too light and required a 50% increase in density to achieve a diagnostic level. What new mAs must be used?

4. A radiograph made using 2.5 mAs must be repeated because it is too light. The quality control technologist requests that you repeat this radiograph and increase the density by 200%. What new mAs would be required?

5. A radiograph was made using the 600-mA station at ¹/₂₀ sec. The radiograph was too dark and you were asked to obtain a radiograph with a 35% reduction in density. What new mAs would be required?

6. The density of the radiograph must be reduced by 30%. The original technique called for 90 kVp at 500 mA for 0.05 sec. What new mAs would be needed and what new time would have to be used if the 500-mA station were *not* to be changed?

7. If the density of a radiograph needed to be increased by 60% and the original technique was 90 kVp at 400 mA for 0.3 sec, what new time would be needed if the 600-mA station were used? State the time in both decimal and fractional form that will afford the most nearly correct mAs.

8. If 90 mAs was used to produce a radiograph and the technologist was told to repeat the film, increasing the density by 100%, what new mAs would be needed?

Introduction to Radiographic Contrast Problems

Contrast is defined as the amount of difference between the blacks and the whites of a radiograph. **Scale of contrast** refers to the number of tonal values from white to black. An image of **short**-scale contrast (high contrast) contains only a few shades of gray, whereas one of **long**-scale contrast (low contrast) contains numerous shades of gray between the white and the black shades, thus providing more information about different densities in the anatomic area being radiographed.

A film with high contrast is intensely black and white and is certainly appealing to the eye, but it is seldom the ideal choice, since diagnostic information can be lost on a radiograph with a short scale of contrast. Low kVp (kilovoltage peak) yields radiographs with high contrast. Higher-kVp radiographs produce images with less contrast and a longer scale of contrast. This usually yields more diagnostic information although the image usually is not the most eye-appealing to radiographers.

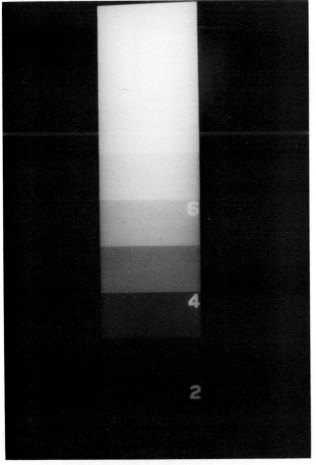
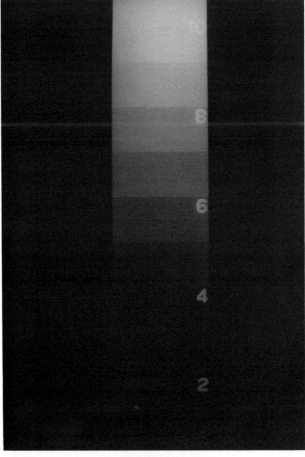

50 kVp (note shorter scale of contrast)　　　　　　　　92 kVp

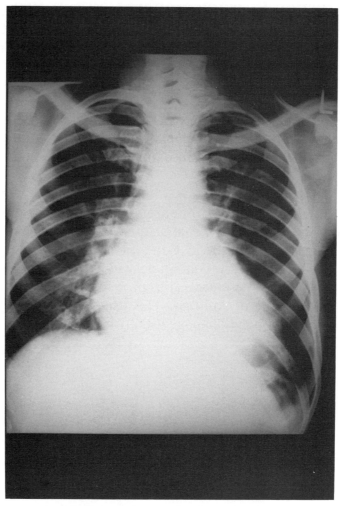

45 kVp (note shorter scale of contrast)

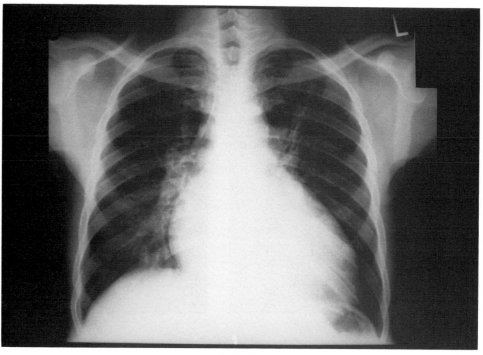

100 kVp

Although it is not generally considered good practice to change the scale of contrast on a radiograph, it is sometimes necessary to obtain more diagnostic information. One of the major factors controlling contrast is kVp. The kVp also affects the density, although it is not generally used for this purpose except in special circumstances where the density must be increased but it is not practical to increase the mA or time. You may see technologists raising or lowering the kVp by 10 to double or halve the density of a radiograph, especially when performing an abdominal series in which the erect view usually requires twice the density of the supine film. This practice is not acceptable, since it is entirely dependent on the original kVp level being used and works well only in the 60 to 80 kVp range. Outside this range, to halve or double the density of the radiograph requires much less than a 10 kVp change below 50 kVp and more than a 10 kVp change above 80 kVp. When altering the kVp is required to change the scale of contrast or to increase or decrease the density, the **15% rule** should be used: a 15% increase or decrease in kVp is equivalent to doubling or halving the density, respectively.

A 15% increase in kVp **lengthens** the **scale** of contrast, thus creating an image with **less** contrast.

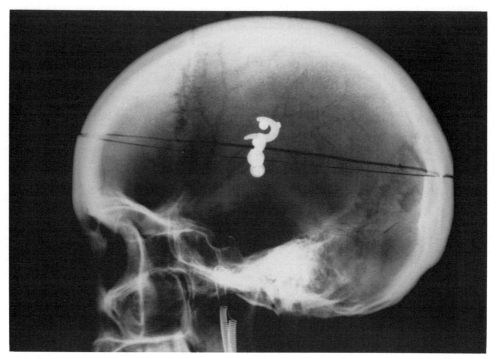

70 kVp

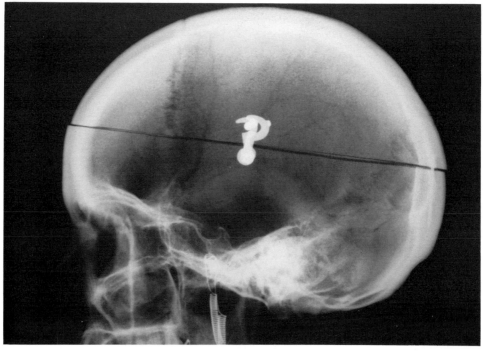

81 kVp (longer scale of contrast [less contrast])

A 15% decrease in kVp **shortens** the **scale** of contrast, thus creating an image with **more** contrast.

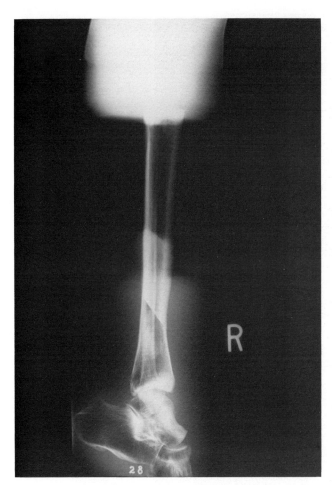

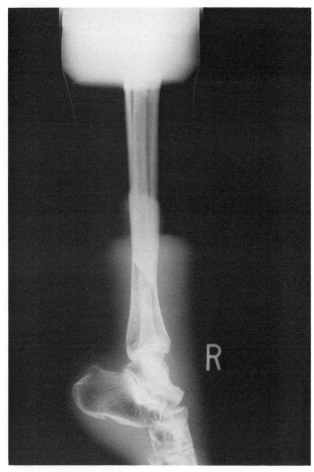

Original at 92 kVp   78 kVp (note increased contrast and therefore better visibility of detail)

A 15% increase in kVp is equivalent to **doubling** the density. To maintain equal density you must cut the mAs in **half**.

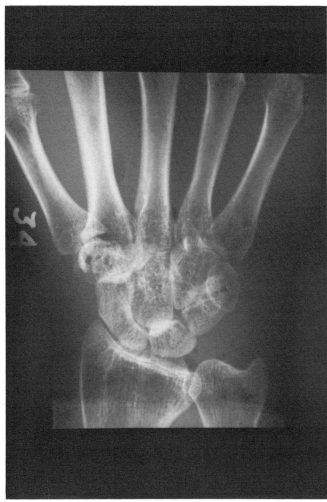

58 kVp at 1.6 mAs (15% increase in kVp)

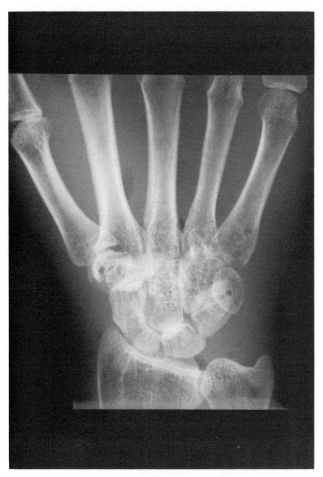 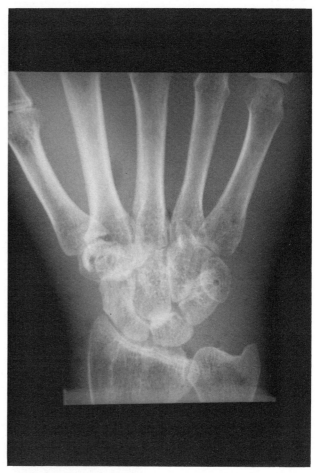

50 kVp at 1.6 mAs (original technique)   58 kVp at 0.8 mAs (15% increase in kVp and half the mAs)

A 15% decrease in kVp is equivalent to cutting the density in **half**. To maintain equal density you must **double** the mAs.

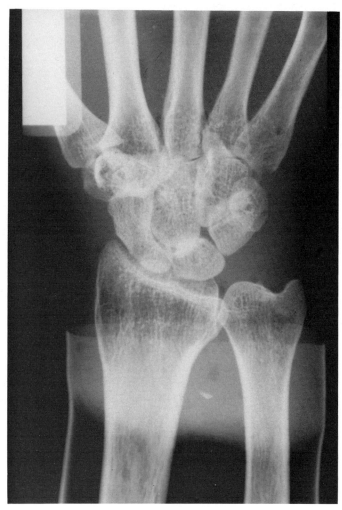

49 kVP at 300 mA for 0.008 s (original technique)

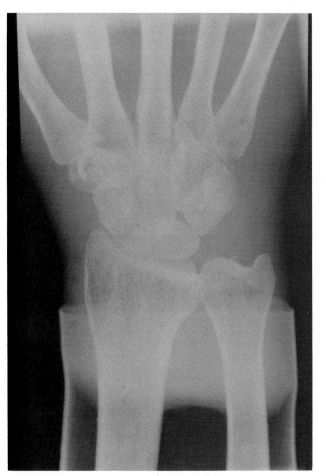

43 kVp at 300 mA for 0.008 s (15% decrease in kVp)

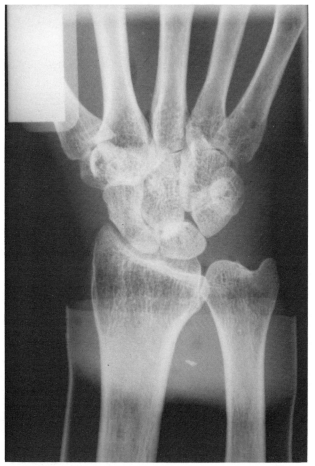

43 kVp at 300 mA for 0.016 s (15% decrease in kVp and twice the mAs)

Example: A radiograph is made using 100 kVp at 40 mAs. It is necessary to double the density but you cannot increase the mA and the patient cannot hold his or her breath any longer. What change in kVp would double the density?

$100 \times 15\% = 100 \times 0.15 = 15$ kVp
$100 + 15 = 115$ kVp

Example: A radiograph needs more contrast to evaluate a possible kidney stone. The original technique was 90 kVp at 300 mA for 0.3 sec. What new technique would better visualize possible kidney stones?

$90 \times 15\% = 100 \times 0.15 = 13.5$ kVp
$90 - 13.5 = 76.5$ kVp

* Note: Because decreasing the kVp by 15% would also cut the density in half, it would be necessary to double the mAs to maintain equal density.

Original mAs = 300 × 0.3 = 90 mAs
New mAs = 90 × 2 = 180 mAs

Using 76 kVp at 180 mAs provides an image with better contrast and a density equal to that of 90 kVp at 90 mAs. What possible mA and time combinations will yield 180 mAs?

300 mA for 0.6 sec = 180 mAs
600 mA for 0.3 sec = 180 mAs

Example: A radiograph exhibits too much contrast, and it is felt that diagnostic information is being lost. The original technique was 68 kVp at 80 mAs. What new technique would provide a longer scale of contrast while maintaining equal density?

68 × 15% = 10.2 kVp
68 + 10.2 = 78.2 kVp

or

68 × 115% = 78.2 kVp

* Note: Because raising the kVp by 15% is equivalent to doubling the density, to maintain equal density you must cut the mAs in half.

80 mAs × ½ = 40 mAs

Using 40 mAs at 78 kVp produces a radiograph with less contrast and a longer scale of contrast but equal density. What mA and time combination would yield 40 mAs?

400 mA for 0.1 sec = 40 mAs
800 mA for 0.05 sec = 40 mAs

Example: A radiograph is made using 80 kVp at 100 mAs for 0.007 sec. The film is too dark and the density must be cut in half. The equipment will not allow the use of a smaller mA station and the time cannot be reduced. What must be done to decrease the density by half?

80 kVp × 15% = 12 kVp
80 kVp − 12 kVp = 68 kVp

or

80 kVp × 85% = 68 kVp

* Note: This decreases the density by 50% without changing the mA or time of exposure.

▼ RADIOGRAPHIC CONTRAST PROBLEMS WORK SHEET ▼

I. Using the 15% rule for changing kVp, fill in the missing information to produce a radiograph that has less contrast (longer scale of contrast) but equal density.

	Original Technique	New Technique
1.	300 mA ³/₂₀ sec 60 kVp	mAs = kVp =
2.	600 mA 0.02 sec 80 kVp	mA = 600 sec = kVp =
3.	50 mAs 500 mA 100 kVp	mA = 500 sec = kVp =
4.	800 mA 0.035 sec 75 kVp	mAs = kVp =
5.	100 mA ¹/₆₀ sec 95 kVp	sec = ¹/₃₀ mA = kVp =

II. Using the 15% rule for changing kVp, fill in the missing information to produce a radiograph that has more contrast (shorter scale of contrast) but equal density.

	Original Technique	New Technique
1.	200 mA ¹/₁₅ sec 120 kVp	mAs = kVp =
2.	25 mA 0.5 sec 90 kVp	mA = 25 sec = kVp =

3.   120 mAs   mA = 400
                 400 mA   sec =
                 110 kVp   kVp =

4.   500 mA   mAs =
                 0.07 sec   kVp =
                 85 kVp

5.   1000 mA   sec = $\frac{1}{60}$
                 $\frac{1}{120}$ mA =
                 115 kVp   kVp =

III. 1. What new mAs and kVp are needed to produce a radiograph with more contrast and half the density if the original technique called for 100 kVp at 600 mA for 0.035 sec?

    2. What new mAs and kVp are needed to produce a radiograph with more contrast and twice the density if the original technique called for 80 kVp at 300 mA for $\frac{3}{20}$ sec?

    3. What new mAs and kVp are needed to produce a radiograph with less contrast and twice the density if the original technique called for 70 kVp at 200 mA for 0.01 sec?

    4. What new mAs and kVp are needed to produce a radiograph with less contrast and half the density if the original technique called for 60 kVp at 400 mA for 0.07 sec?

Introduction to Radiographic Screen Conversion

Sometimes it is necessary to adjust technique to compensate for a change in screen speed. As with a change in grids, the usual method of compensating for a change in screen speed is to adjust mAs. (Some department protocols may direct the radiographer to add or subtract a specified amount of kVp when changing from one screen speed to another.) The required change in mAs can be calculated by assigning a correction factor for each of the common speeds of screens, the par speed screen being the standard. The standard screen (par speed) is the one on which all correction factors are based.

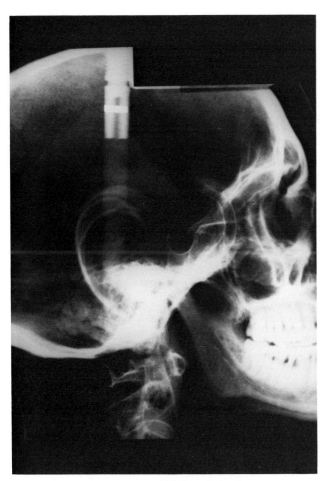

200-speed system 70 kVp at 2.5 mAs

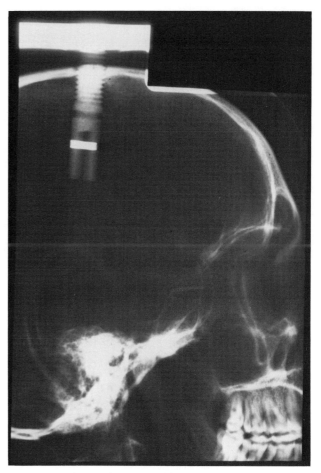

400-speed system 70 kVp at 2.5 mAs

* Note: It should be noted that changes in screen speed cause changes in the scale of contrast as well as the density of a radiograph. As screen speed increases so do contrast and density. However, some recorded detail of definition is lost. Contrast and density are lost as screen speed is reduced, but recorded detail or definition improves.

Direct exposure/cardboard holder	50 × mAs
Detail/50-speed system	2 × mAs
Par/100-speed system	1 × mAs
(calcium tungstate)	
High speed/200-speed system	½ × mAs
(calcium tungstate)	
Rare earth (200)-speed system	½ × mAs
(400)-speed system	¼ × mAs
(800)-speed system	⅛ × mAs

* Note: These factors may vary with manufacturers.

Example: If a radiograph is made using 60 mAs with a 100-speed system, what mAs would be needed if a 200-speed system were used?

Conversion factor $\dfrac{\text{New}}{\text{Old}} = \dfrac{½}{1} = ½$

$60 × ½ = 30$ mAs

Example: If 30 mAs is the normal technique used with rare earth screens (400 system) and a 200-speed system must be used, what mAs is required?

Conversion factor $\dfrac{\text{New}}{\text{Old}} = \dfrac{½}{¼} = 2$

$30 × 2 = 60$ mAs

▼ SCREEN CONVERSION WORK SHEET ▼

1. If 80 mAs is needed for a particular radiograph using a 100-speed system, what mAs would be needed using a 400 rare earth system?

2. If 2½ mAs is used with a 200-speed system, what mAs would be needed if an 800-speed system is used?

3. If 70 mAs is the normal technique used with rare earth screens (400 system) and a 100-speed system had to be used, what mAs would be required?

4. If a radiograph is made using 90 mAs with detail screens, what mAs would be needed if a 200-speed rare earth system were used?

5. If a radiograph is made using 30 mAs with a 100-speed system, what mAs would be needed if a 200-speed system is used?

6. If 50 mAs is the normal technique used with a 200-speed system and a 100-speed system had to be used, what mAs would be required?

7. If 3 mAs is adequate for a radiograph exposed using an 800 rare earth system, what mAs would be necessary if a 400 rare earth system were used?

8. If 20 mAs is needed to adequately expose a radiograph with a 200 rare earth system, what mAs would be needed with an 800 rare earth system?

9. If an exposure is made using 1.5 mAs with a 200-speed system, what mAs would be needed if the radiographer were asked to use a direct exposure technique?

10. If 21 mAs is needed for a radiograph using a 400-speed rare earth system, what mAs would be needed with a 200-speed system?

Grid Ratio

A grid used in radiography is formed from a series of very thin lead strips separated by interspace material. Grids are classified according to **grid ratio,** which is the relationship between the height of the lead strips and the distance between them.

$$\text{Grid ratio} = \frac{\text{Height of lead strip } (h)}{\text{Distance between strips } (w)}$$

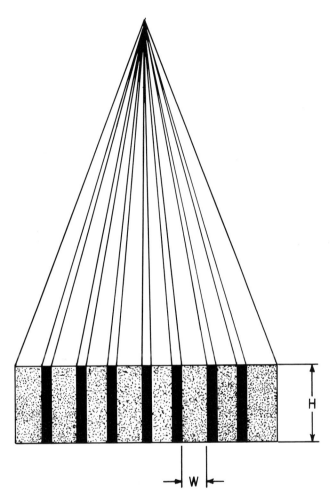

Example: If the height of the lead strips is 1.6 mm and the width between the strips is 0.1 mm, the ratio of the grid is _____ .

$$\frac{1.6}{0.1} = 16$$

Grid ratio = 16 : 1

▼ GRID RATIO WORK SHEET ▼

1. What is the ratio of a grid if the height of the lead strips is 1.2 mm and the distance between them is 0.1 mm?

2. What is the ratio of a grid if the height of the lead strips is 0.8 mm and the distance between them is 0.1 mm?

3. What is the ratio of a grid if the height of the lead strips is 0.5 mm and the distance between them is 0.1 mm?

4. What is the ratio of a grid if the height of the lead strips is 0.6 mm and the distance between them is 0.1 mm?

5. What is the ratio of a grid if the height of the lead strips is 1.0 mm and the distance between them is 0.1 mm?

Introduction to Grid Conversion

Grids are used to improve contrast, especially when radiographing any part that measures 10 cm or greater. The grid is composed of lead strips that absorb secondary radiation that would otherwise fog the image. Depending on the ratio (height of lead strips to the distance between them) and frequency (number of lead strips or lines per inch), a grid can absorb up to 90% of the secondary radiation that otherwise would reach the film. It is essential that the radiographer make adjustments in technical factors to compensate for this absorption of radiation. Although one can alter the kVp, the usual method of adjustment is to change the mAs, which is dependent on the grid ratio. Some department protocols may direct the radiographer to add or subtract a specified amount of kVp when changing from one type of grid to another (these factors change slightly if stationary grids are used). One of the easiest methods used to calculate the change in technique required by the addition of a grid (or by changing from one grid ratio to another) is to assign a correction factor value to each grid as follows:

$$
\begin{array}{ll}
\text{No grid} & = 1 \\
5:1 & = 2 \\
6:1 & = 3 \\
8:1 & = 4 \\
12:1 & = 5 \\
16:1 & = 6
\end{array}
$$

To determine the new mAs required because of a change in a grid, the correction factor of the new grid is divided by the correction factor of the old grid, and the quotient is multiplied by the original mAs. The formula is as follows:

$$\text{New mAs} = \text{Old mAs} \times \frac{\text{New grid correction factor}}{\text{Old grid correction factor}}$$

or

$$mAs_2 = mAs_1 \times \frac{G_2}{G_1}$$

Example: The technique chart for a particular examination recommends using 90 mAs and a 12:1 grid. What new mAs would be needed using a 6:1 grid?

$$mAs_2 = mAs_1 \times \frac{G_2}{G_1}$$

$$mAs_2 = 90 \times \tfrac{3}{5}$$
$$mAs_2 = 54 \text{ mAs}$$

Example: If 50 mAs is an appropriate technique for obtaining a radiograph of a particular patient using a 6 : 1 grid, what new mAs would be required using a 16 : 1 grid to obtain a radiograph with equal density?

$$mAs_2 = mAs_1 \times \frac{G_2}{G_1}$$
$$mAs_2 = 50 \times \frac{6}{3}$$
$$mAs_2 = 100 \text{ mAs}$$

* Note: After working this problem it should be noted that increasing the grid ratio causes a decrease in density. It should also be noted that this loss in density, due to less scattered radiation reaching the film, causes an increase in contrast or a shorter scale of contrast.

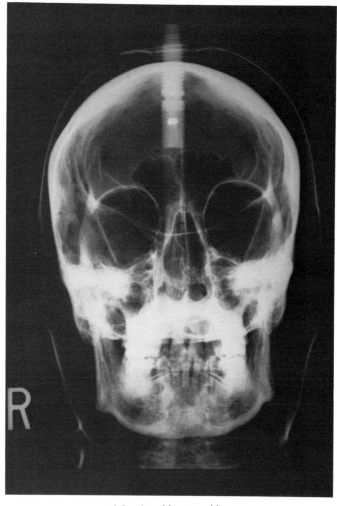

0.8 mAs without a grid

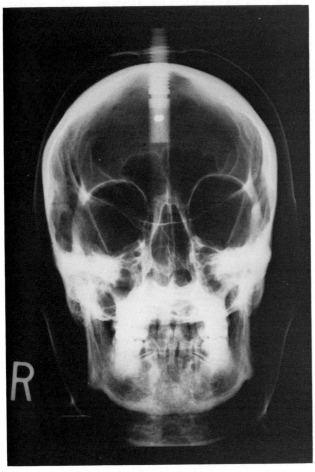

1 mAs with a 6 : 1 grid

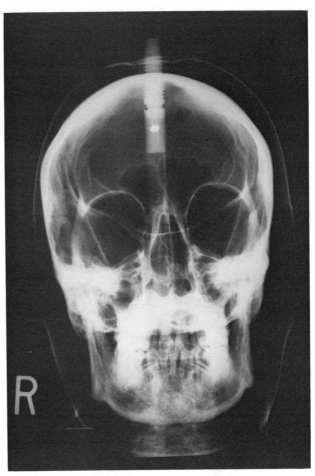

1.6 mAs with an 8 : 1 grid

▼ GRID CONVERSION WORK SHEET ▼

1. If 30 mAs is the technique needed to obtain a radiograph using an 8 : 1 grid, what mAs would be required if a 12 : 1 grid is used?

2. If a radiograph made using a 6 : 1 grid had to be repeated without a grid, what mAs would be needed if the original mAs was 15?

3. If 300 mA for $\frac{1}{15}$ second is used to expose a radiograph made without a grid, what mAs would be needed using a 6 : 1 grid?

4. If a radiograph is made using a 16 : 1 grid with 120 mAs, what mAs would be needed with a 12 : 1 grid?

5. If 10 mAs is needed with a 5 : 1 grid, what mAs would be needed with a 12 : 1 grid?

6. If the technique for a radiograph made using a 12 : 1 grid required 60 mAs, what mAs would be needed if a 5 : 1 grid is used?

7. If 150 mAs is needed with a 16 : 1 grid, what mAs would be needed with an 8 : 1 grid?

8. If 2.5 mAs is needed with a 5 : 1 grid, what mAs would be needed with a 16 : 1 grid?

9. If 600 mA for 0.35 sec is needed to expose a radiograph using a 16 : 1 grid, what mAs would be needed with an 8 : 1 grid?

10. If 200 mA for $\frac{1}{40}$ sec is used to expose a radiograph without a grid, what mAs would be needed with a 16 : 1 grid?

Geometric Unsharpness

It is sometimes necessary to measure the amount of geometric un-sharpness on a radiographic image. This unsharpness, commonly referred to as **penumbra**, is due to the divergence of the x-ray beam and can be predicted and controlled somewhat by the use of a proper combination of focal spot size (FSS), focus–object distance (FOD), and object–film distance (OFD). Some textbooks refer to object–film distance as object–image receptor distance (OID). Although it is beyond the scope of this text to explore all of the possibilities, it is important to learn how to use the following algebraic formula to determine unsharpness.

$$\text{Geometric unsharpness} = \frac{\text{Focal spot size} \times \text{Object–film distance}}{\text{Focus–object distance}}$$

or

$$= \frac{\text{FSS} \times \text{OFD}}{\text{FOD}}$$

* Note: The source–image receptor distance (SID) equals the sum of the OFD and the FOD.

Example: Determine the amount of geometric unsharpness if the focal spot size (FSS) is 2.5 mm, the OFD is 8 in, and the FOD is 32 in.

$$x = \frac{2.5 \times 8}{32}$$

$x = {}^{20}\!/_{32}$

$x = {}^{5}\!/_{8}$ or 0.625

This figure represents the amount of geometric unsharpness present when these factors are used. One can infer from this problem that the FFD was 40 in (OFD + FOD = SID).

One very obvious method of reducing unsharpness is to **increase** the total source–image receptor distance, thus increasing the FOD, which decreases the amount of unsharpness.

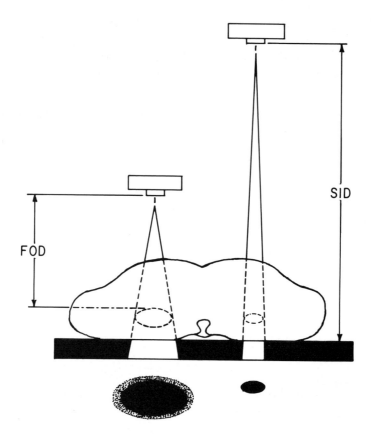

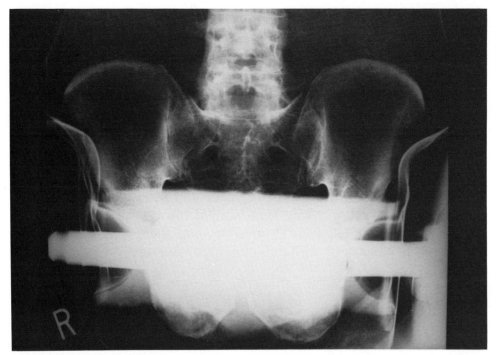

40-in SID

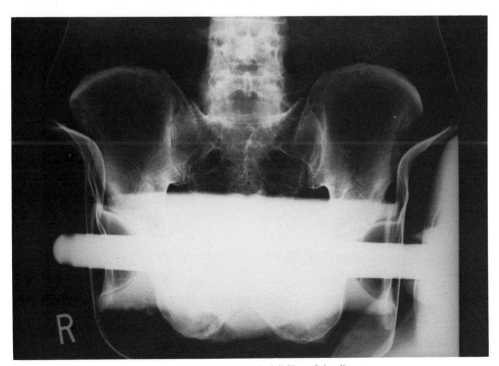

60-in SID (note increased visibility of detail)

If the SID were increased from 40 in to 48 in, thus increasing the FOD to 40 in, the unsharpness would be reduced to:

$$x = \frac{2.5 \times 8}{40}$$
$$x = {}^{20}\!/_{40}$$
$$x = {}^{1}\!/_{2} \quad \text{or} \quad 0.05$$

* Note: This is a slight decrease in the amount of unsharpness.

After working the following work sheet you should realize that to improve radiographic quality you should always use the smallest practical FSS, the least OFD possible, and the maximum SID or FOD that is consistent with equipment capabilities.

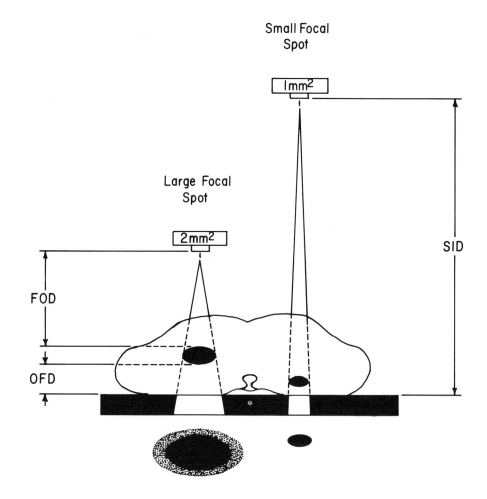

▼ GEOMETRIC UNSHARPNESS
WORK SHEET ▼

Determine the amount of geometric unsharpness that would be present on a radiograph produced using the following factors:

1. FSS = 1.5
    OFD = 3 in
    FOD = 32 in

2. FSS = 3
    OFD = 4.5 in
    FOD = 31.5 in

3. FSS = 2
    OFD = 2 in
    SID = 44 in
    (Remember to determine FOD before working formula.)

4. FSS = 1
    FOD = 38 in
    SID = 48 in
    (Remember to determine OFD before working formula.)

5. FSS = 3.5
    OFD = 4 in
    FOD = 68 in

6. FSS = 2.5
    OFD = 6 in
    FOD = 34 in

7. FSS = 3
    OFD = 12 in
    SID = 60 in

8. FSS = 1
    OFD = 12 in
    SID = 72 in

9. FSS = 1
    OFD = 2 in
    SID = 72 in

10. FSS = 2
    FOD = 70 in
    SID = 72 in

Determine how the following changes will affect the quality or resolution of the radiographic image: A, decrease; B, increase; or C, no change.

11. Increase in OFD

12. Increase in SID

13. Increase in FSS

14. Decrease in SID

15. Decrease in OFD

16. Decrease in FSS

17. Proportional increase in SID and OFD

18. Proportional increase in OFD and FOD

Now that you have finished this work sheet, go back and analyze the results of increasing the SID and the effect it has on image unsharpness. Note Problems 7 and 8, in which not only was the SID **increased** but the FSS was **decreased,** resulting in a dramatic reduction in image unsharpness. In Problems 9 and 10 notice how an **increase** in FSS **increases** the amount of image unsharpness. By noting the effects of these changes now, you can begin to see some of the important relationships that affect radiographic quality and learn early in your training how to adjust various factors to improve the quality of your finished radiographs. These concepts are illustrated in the following four radiographs.

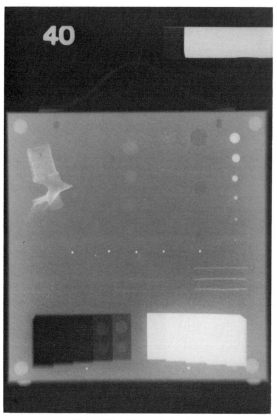

40-in SID with small focal spot

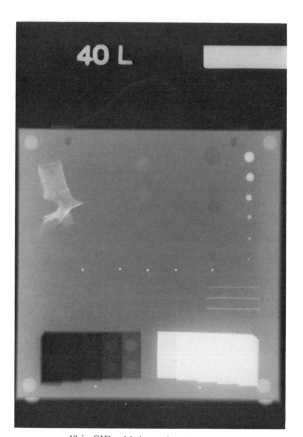

40-in SID with large focal spot

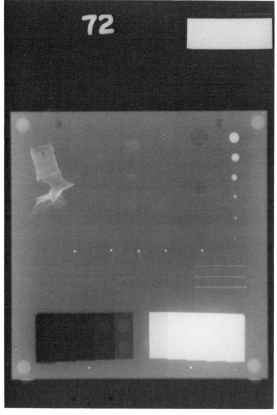

72-in SID with small focal spot

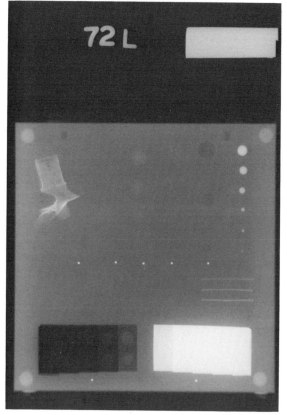

72-in SID with large focal spot

Magnification Unsharpness

All radiographic images possess some magnification unsharpness, or distortion. This causes a loss in image resolution, or quality. To determine the true size of an object or its projected image, one can use the following proportion:

$$\frac{\text{Object size (OS)}}{\text{Image size (IS)}} = \frac{\text{Focus–object distance}}{\text{Source–image receptor distance}}$$

or

$$\frac{\text{OS}}{\text{IS}} = \frac{\text{FOD}}{\text{SID}}$$

Example: If an object measures 2 in and the FOD is 38 in while the FFD is 40 in, what will be the size of the projected image on the radiograph?

$$\frac{2 \text{ in}}{x} = \frac{38 \text{ in}}{40 \text{ in}}$$
$$38x \text{ in} = 80 \text{ in}^2$$
$$x = 2.1 \text{ in (size of projected image)}$$

It is also possible to predict the amount of magnification of an image projected onto a radiograph by using the following formula:

$$\text{Magnification factor (MF)} = \frac{\text{SID}}{\text{FOD}}$$

Example: Using the figures from the example above, what will be the magnification factor for an object using a 38-in FOD and a 40-in SID?

$$\text{MF} = {}^{40}\!/_{38}$$
$$\text{MF} = 1.05$$

* Note: The projected image will be 1.05 times as large as the actual object, or 1.05 × 2 in = 2.1 in.

To determine the percent of magnification, use this formula:

$$\text{Magnification (\%)} = \frac{\text{OFD}}{\text{FOD}} \times 100$$

Example: Using the factors from the examples above, what is the percent of magnification?

To determine the OFD:

OFD = SID − FOD
OFD = 40 − 38 = 2 in

$$\text{Magnification} = \frac{2}{38} \times 100$$
$$\frac{200 \text{ in}}{38 \text{ in}} = 5.26\%$$

If the actual object measured 2 in and the percent of magnification was 5.26% you could predict that the image size projected onto the radiograph would be 2.1 in.

Image size = Object size + % Magnification

IS = 2 + (2 × 5.26%)
IS = 2 + 0.1 = 2.1 in

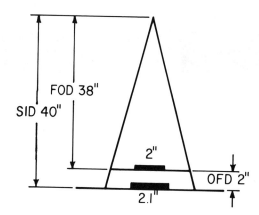

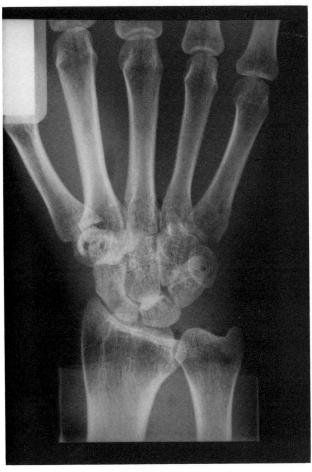

½-in OFD (object–film distance)

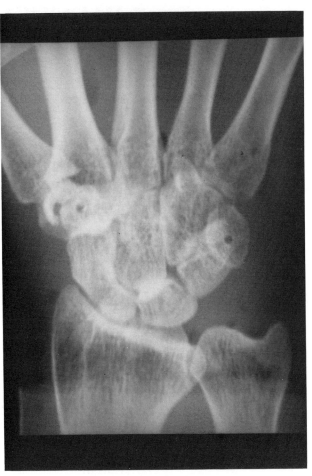

8-in OFD (note blurring of image)

▼ MAGNIFICATION UNSHARPNESS WORK SHEET ▼

1. Determine the size of the projected image of an object that measures 7 in if using an FFD of 44 in and an FOD of 40 in.

2. Determine the size of the projected image of an object that measures 3.5 in if using an FFD of 36 in and an FOD of 30 in.

3. Determine the size of the projected image of an object that measures 12 in if using an FFD of 40 in and an FOD of 34 inches.

4. Determine the size of the projected image of an object that measures 8 in if using an FFD of 48 in and an FOD of 44 in.

5. Determine the magnification factor if the FFD is 40 in and the FOD is 36 in.

6. Determine the magnification factor if the FFD is 72 in and the FOD is 68 in.

7. Determine the magnification factor if the FFD is 60 in and the FOD is 54 in.

8. Determine the percent of magnification if the OFD is 3 in and the FOD is 41 in.

9. Determine the percent of magnification if the OFD is 6 in and the FOD is 30 in.

10. Determine the percent of magnification if the OFD is 2 in and the FOD is 40 in.

11. What will be the projected image size of a 10-in object if the OFD is 2 in and the FOD is 38 in?

12. What will be the projected image size of a 4-in object if the OFD is 4 in and the FOD is 40 in?

13. What will be the projected image size of a 15-in object if the OFD is 3 in and the FOD is 33 in?

14. What will be the projected image size of a 25.4-cm object if the OFD is 5.08 cm and the FOD is 96.52 cm?

15. Convert the answer to Problem 14 into inches (2.54 cm = 1 in).

16. If the FFD is 72 in and the OFD is 2 in, what is the percentage of magnification?

17. If the FFD is 60 in and the FOD is 56 in, what will be the size of the image projected onto the radiograph if the object is 15 in?

18. If an object measures 38 cm and the FFD is 40 in, the size of the projected image will be what percentage larger if the OFD is 6 in?

19. What is the magnification factor for an object if the FFD is 72 in and the OFD is 2 in?

20. Determine the true size of an object if the image size is 12 in using an FFD of 40 in and an FOD of 36 in.

Graphs

A graph is a pictorial representation of numeric values represented as positions in a plane. Using this technique, the often complicated relationship between two specific quantities can be expressed as a curved or straight line.

Most graphs are composed of two **axes:** a horizontal, or **x axis,** and a vertical, or **y axis.** The point at which these two axes meet is called the **origin.** Each point on a graph is precisely defined by a pair of **coordinates.** The first number of the pair represents the distance along the x axis. The second number of the pair represents the distance along the y axis. For example, on the graph below, the coordinates of point A are (7,6) and the coordinates of point B are (10,11).

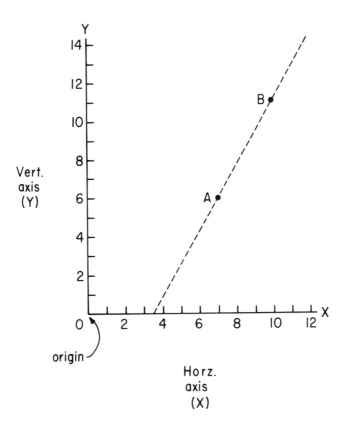

The x and y axes can represent any type of quantity. For example, a practical problem in radiologic technology is the effect of varying amounts of mAs on the film density (darkening) of the radiograph. In the following graph, the x axis represents mAs and the y axis represents density. For any mAs setting the resulting density can be determined. Conversely, to achieve a specific density the required mAs can be calculated.

Example: Using an mAs of 60 results in what film density?

To solve this problem, first go along the *x* axis to an mAs of 60. From it draw a perpendicular line that intersects the curve. Then draw a line perpendicular to this point to intersect the *y* axis. The number at this point is 1.2, which represents the resulting density.

Example: To achieve a density of 0.8 what mAs is required?

To solve this problem, first go along the *y* axis to a density of 0.8. Draw a perpendicular line to the right that intersects the curve. From this point, draw a perpendicular line downward to intersect the *x* axis. The number at this point is 30, which represents the mAs required to achieve this film density.

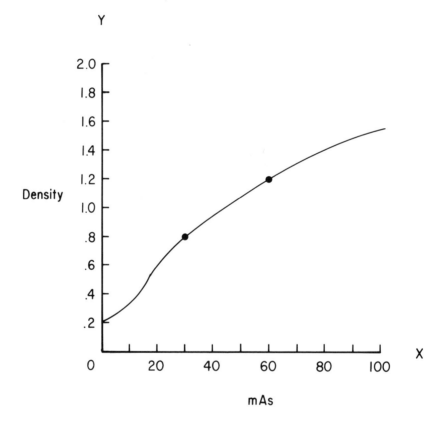

One common use of graphs in radiologic technology is the tube-rating chart that indicates the maximum safe exposure time for any selected combination of kVp and mA for a single exposure and a relatively cool tube.

Example: Using 400 mA, what is the maximum exposure time in seconds when using a kVp of 100?

To solve this problem, first go up the *y* axis to 100 kVp. Draw a perpendicular line that intersects the curve marked 400 mA. From this point draw a perpendicular line that extends to the *x* axis. The number at the point of intersection is 3 sec, which represents the maximum exposure time.

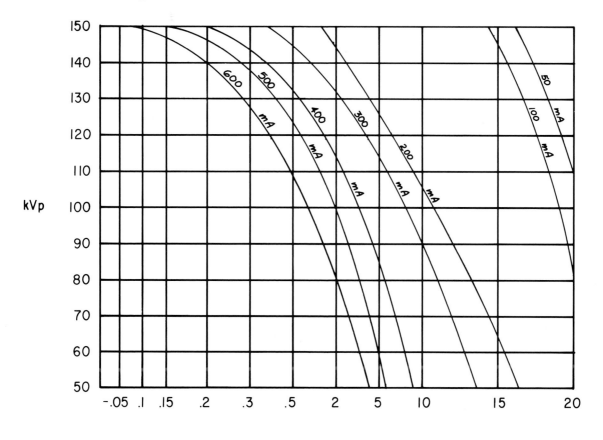

At times, radiographers also must deal with graphs based on a **logarithmic** scale. Although it is beyond the scope of this book to discuss logarithms in depth, it should be mentioned that sensitometric or characteristic curves plotted on a logarithmic scale are frequently used to assign numeric values to such important radiographic factors as contrast, density, and exposure.

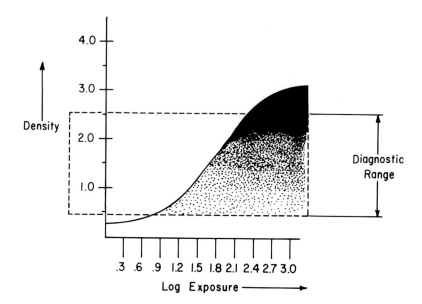

▼ GRAPH WORK SHEET ▼

Using the graph below determine the missing factor for the exposures listed.

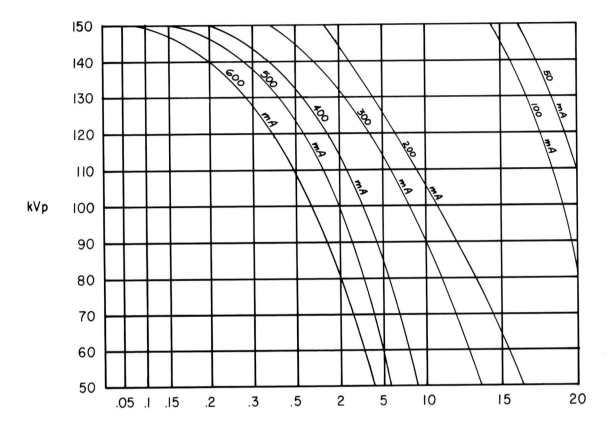

Seconds

	kVp	mA	Maximum Exposure Time
1.	90	300	_____
2.	70	600	_____
3.	80	200	_____
4.	____	500	0.15 sec
5.	____	100	20 sec
6.	100	____	2 sec

Conventional Units and Système International Conversions

Conversion of conventional to Système International (SI) units and vice versa is often necessary when determining radiation dosimetry. The terms used for conventional units are these:

Roentgen (R) — an expression of exposure
Radiation absorbed dose (rad) — the energy absorbed dose
Radiation equivalent man (rem) — an expression of the biologic dose in humans
Curie (Ci) — a unit of radioactivity

Certain organizations and textbooks have adopted SI units. Students will use the following conversions in radiation protection and biology classes.

$$1 \text{ R} \times (2.58 \times 10^{-4}) = 1 \text{ coulomb per kilogram (C/kg)}$$
$$1 \text{ rad} \times 0.01 = 1 \text{ gray (Gy)}$$
$$1 \text{ rem} \times 0.01 = 1 \text{ sievert (Sv)}$$
$$1 \text{ Ci} \times (3.7 \times 10^{10}) = 1 \text{ becquerel (Bq)}$$

To convert from SI units to conventional units, multiply or divide the SI units by the conversion factors shown above.

Example: 40 rad is equivalent to _____ gray.

$$40 \times 0.01 = 0.4 \text{ Gy}$$

Example: 500 rem is equivalent to _____ sievert.

$$500 \times 0.01 = 5 \text{ Sv}$$

Example: 50 Sv is equivalent to _____ rem.

$$50 \div 0.01 = 5000 \text{ rem}$$

▼ CONVENTIONAL UNITS AND SYSTÈME INTERNATIONAL CONVERSIONS WORK SHEET ▼

I. Convert the following quantities to SI units:

1. 200 rad

2. 5 rem

3. 0.05 rem

4. 17 rad

5. 5 R

II. Convert the following quantities to conventional units:

1. 10 Sv

2. 40 Gy

3. 500 Gy

4. 0.01 Sv

5. 10 Bq

Physics Formulas

Although a detailed discussion of physics is beyond the scope of this book, many formulas in your physics classes require you to utilize your knowledge of basic algebra. The following list contains some (certainly not all) of the formulas you will be required to use, as well as brief descriptive statements. You should refer to your physics text for further explanation.

Ohm's Law

In an electrical circuit, the current (I, in amperes) equals the potential difference (in volts) divided by the resistance (R, in ohms). This is expressed algebraically:

$$I = \frac{V}{R}$$

This is the same as

$$V = IR \quad \text{or} \quad R = \frac{V}{I}$$

If any two of these values are known, the third can be easily found by simply substituting in the equation and solving for the unknown.

Example: If 1 ampere (A) of current flows through a conductor with 5 ohms of resistance, the voltage will be _____.

$$\text{Voltage} = 1A \times 5$$
$$= 5 \text{ V}$$

Heat Units

The heat storage capacity of the anode is measured in heat units (hu), which for single-phase power supplies equals the product of the current (in mA), kVp, and time (in seconds). This can be expressed in the following formula:

$$\text{hu} = \text{mA} \times \text{kVp} \times \text{sec}$$

* Note: When using three-phase 6-pulse equipment you must multiply the original formula by 1.35. When using three-phase 12-pulse equipment you must multiply the original formula by 1.41.

Example: 100 kVp at 600 mA for 0.05 sec creates _____ heat units.

$$100 \text{ kVp} \times 600 \text{ mA} \times 0.05 = 60{,}000 \times 0.05 = 3000 \text{ hu}$$

Transformer Laws

A transformer is an electromagnetic device that changes alternating current from high voltage to low voltage and vice versa. The ratio of the voltages in the primary and secondary circuits is proportional to the number of turns in their respective coils. This can be expressed as:

$$\frac{V_p}{V_s} = \frac{N_p}{N_s}$$

N_p = Number of turns in the primary coil
N_s = Number of turns in the secondary coil
V_p = Voltage in the primary circuit
V_s = Voltage in the secondary circuit

Example: The primary coil of a transformer has 100 turns and the secondary coil has 20,000. What is the potential difference of the secondary coil if the primary has 200 volts?

$$\frac{100}{20{,}000} = \frac{200}{x}$$
$$100x = 4{,}000{,}000$$
$$x = 40{,}000 \text{ volts}$$

Because a transformer cannot create energy, an increase in voltage must be accompanied by a corresponding decrease in current, so the product of the voltage and current (I) in the two circuits must be equal. This can be written as follows:

$$V_p I_p = V_s I_s$$

V_p = Voltage in the primary coil
I_p = Current in the primary coil
V_s = Voltage in the secondary coil
I_s = Current in the secondary coil

Example: Using the information from the previous example you can determine the current in the secondary coil if you know the current in the primary one. In this example the primary current is 20 amperes; therefore the current in the secondary will be _____ amperes (A) or _____ milliamperes (mA).

$$100 \times 20 = 20,000 \times x$$
$$2,000 = 20,000x$$
$$0.1 \text{ A} = x$$

or

$$100 \text{ mA} = x$$

Power Rule

The power rule states that in an electric circuit the energy used per second (power, expressed in watts) is simply the product of the current (I, in amperes) and voltage. Thus:

$$P \text{ (in watts)} = IV$$

Example: If the voltage is 100 and the current is 200 amperes, the power will be _____ watts.

$$P = 200 \times 100$$
$$P = 20,000 \text{ watts}$$

The power of an electric current is decreased by the amount of heat produced in the circuit. This power loss (in heat production per second) can be calculated in terms of the resistance (which remains constant regardless of the current or voltage). Inserting Ohm's law $\left(I = \dfrac{V}{R}, \text{ or } V = IR\right)$ from page 124 into the above equation:

$$P = I \times IR$$
$$\text{Power loss} = I^2R$$

Example: If a circuit has 200 A of current and 1 ohm resistance, the power loss would be _____ watts.

$$P = 200^2 \times 1$$
$$P = 40,000 \times 1$$
$$P = 40,000 \text{ watts}$$

Kinetic Energy

The kinetic energy (ability to do work, expressed in joules) of a moving body equals half its mass (in kilograms) times the square of the velocity (in meters per second). This can be written:

$$KE = \frac{1}{2} mv^2$$

Series and Parallel Circuits

In a *series* circuit the component parts are arranged end-to-end, so that the current passes consecutively through each part. The total resistance of the whole circuit equals the sum of the separate resistances.

$$R = r_1 + r_2 + r_3 \ldots + r_x$$

$$R = \text{total resistance}$$
$$r_1, r_2, r_3 = \text{resistances of the parts of the circuit}$$

Example: In a series circuit of three elements with resistances of 6 ohms, 3 ohms, and 1 ohm, respectively, the total resistance of the circuit is _____ ohms.

$$6 + 3 + 1 = 10 \text{ ohms}$$

In a *parallel* circuit, the **reciprocal** of the total resistance (R) equals the sum of the reciprocals of the separate resistances (r_1, r_2, r_3, . . . , r_x).

Example: In a parallel circuit of three elements with resistances of 6 ohms, 3 ohms, and 1 ohm, respectively, the total resistance of the circuit is _____ ohms.

$$\frac{1}{R} = \frac{1}{6} + \frac{1}{3} + \frac{1}{1}$$

$$\frac{1}{R} = \frac{1}{6} + \frac{2}{6} + \frac{6}{6}$$

$$\frac{1}{R} = \frac{9}{6}$$

$$R = \frac{6}{9} = \frac{2}{3} \text{ ohm}$$

Energy Conversion

X-rays are produced by energy conversion when fast-moving electrons from the filament of the x-ray tube interact with the tungsten anode (target). The increase in the kinetic energy (E) of the electron in passing across the voltage (V) can be expressed:

$$E \text{ (in joules)} = e\text{V}$$

$$e = \text{electron charge } (1.6 \times 10^{-9} \text{ coulomb})$$

Propagation of X-Rays

To describe the propagation of electromagnetic radiation through space in the form of *waves,* the velocity (V) equals the wavelength (λ) times the frequency (v):

$$V = \lambda v$$

Since electromagnetic radiation always travels at the speed of light (c), which is 186,000 miles/sec or 3×10^8 meters/sec, the above equation can be written:

$$c = \lambda v$$

To describe the propagation of electromagnetic radiation through space in the form of *particles* (bundles of energy called quanta or photons), the photon energy (E) equals the frequency (v) times Planck's constant (h):

$$E = \text{h}v$$

$$\text{h} = 4.13 \times 10^{-8} \text{ keV/sec}$$

Combining the wave and particle aspects of electromagnetic radiation produces the classic formula:

$$E = \frac{\text{hc}}{\lambda}$$

Since the product of the velocity of light (c) and Planck's constant (h) is 12.4 when the unit of energy is keV and the wavelength is measured in Angströms, the classic final equation describing the relation between energy (E) and wavelength (λ) is:

$$E = \frac{12.4}{\lambda}$$

PRACTICAL APPLICATIONS

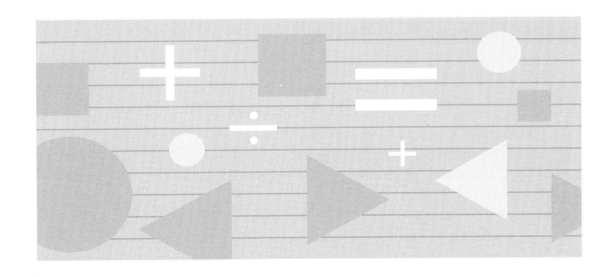

▼ OBJECTIVES SECTION THREE ▼

After completing this section, the student will be able to perform radiographic calculations necessary to adjust technical factors for the variations that occur in all radiology departments as well as to work required classroom calculations.

Practical Problems

1. A radiograph is made using 90 kVp at 300 mA for 0.035 sec. The quality control technologist asks that you repeat this film using 40% less mAs. What new time would be needed if you are to continue to use the 300 mA station?

2. You radiograph the lumbar spine of an elderly woman and note that she has advanced osteoporosis with substantial calcium loss. The film fails to demonstrate the needed diagnostic information because of the lack of contrast. What change in the technique would you make if you originally used 90 kVp at 150 mAs?

3. You made a cross-table lateral radiograph of a broken femur employing a 6 : 1 stationary grid and using 74 kVp at 300 mA for 0.05 sec. The orthopedic physician applies a long leg splint to the patient and requests that you repeat the film. Another technologist has taken the 6 : 1 grid on a portable and you must use an 8 : 1 grid for your follow-up film. What new technique would be needed to provide the same radiographic density?

4. You made a portable chest radiograph of a recumbent patient and are now asked to repeat the examination with the patient in the erect position. Your original technique was 86 kVp and 1.6 mAs at a 44-in distance. When you repeat the study in the erect position you will be using a 68-in distance. What new mAs would be needed to obtain equal density?

5. You make an AP abdominal radiograph of a patient who is unable to hold his breath. Because of excessive motion you must repeat the film. Your original technique was 80 kVp at 300 mA for 0.15 sec. How would you change this technique to try to eliminate the motion while maintaining the same density?

6. You made a PA chest radiograph of a patient using 120 kVp at 1.125 mAs. The radiologist requests a repeat PA chest film with the kVp not to exceed 80. What new technique would provide the radiologist with a film of the same density using no more than 80 kVp?

7. You are told to increase the density of a radiograph by 50%. Your original technique was 90 kVp at 600 mA for 0.05 sec. What new technique would be used if you were to change only the time, leaving the mA and kVp the same?

8. A radiograph is produced with a 6 : 1 grid using 70 kVp at 200 mA for 0.03 sec. You are asked to repeat the examination using an 8 : 1 grid. What new technique would be needed?

9. A radiograph is produced with an 8 : 1 grid using 90 kVp at 400 mA for 0.08 sec. You are asked to repeat the examination using a 12 : 1 grid. What new technique would be needed?

10. A radiograph is produced with a 16 : 1 grid using 100 kVp at 800 mA for 0.02 sec. You are asked to repeat the examination using a 12 : 1 grid. What new technique would be needed?

11. A radiograph is produced with a 5 : 1 grid using 70 kVp at 800 mA for 0.02 sec. You are asked to repeat the examination using a 6 : 1 grid. What new technique would be needed?

12. A radiograph is produced with a 16 : 1 grid using 120 kVp at 600 mA for ¹⁄₁₀ sec. You are asked to repeat the examination using only 100 kVp. What new technique would be needed?

13. A radiograph is produced with a 12 : 1 grid using 100 kVp at 600 mA for ¹⁄₃₀ sec. You are asked to repeat the examination using 80 kVp. What new technique would be needed?

14. A radiograph is produced with an 8 : 1 grid using 80 kVp at 300 mA for 1.5 sec. You are asked to repeat the examination using 100 kVp. What new technique would be needed?

15. A radiograph is produced with a 6 : 1 grid using 70 kVp at 100 mA for ¹⁄₁₅ sec. You are asked to repeat the examination using 80 kVp. What new technique would be needed?

16. A radiograph is made using 100-speed screens with 40 mAs. What new mAs would be needed if slow-speed screens were substituted?

17. A radiograph is made using 10 mAs and 50-speed (detail) screens. What new mAs would be needed if 100-speed screens were substituted?

18. A radiograph is made using 200-speed screens, and the radiologist requests that you repeat the study using 50-speed (detail) screens. If your original technique called for 3.5 mAs, what new mAs would be needed?

19. A radiograph made with 200-speed screens must be repeated using 100-speed screens. If your original technique called for 5 mAs, what new mAs would be needed?

20. You are using 10 mAs with 100-speed screens and decide to repeat the study using 200-speed screens to help eliminate motion. What new mAs would be needed?

In your radiographic exposure class you were asked to identify which technique in each problem will give you the radiograph with the greatest density.

					Distance	
21.	A.	70 kVp	500 mA	1/10 sec	40″ SID	6 : 1 grid
	B.	75 kVp	300 mA	1/15 sec	44″ SID	5 : 1 grid
	C.	80 kVp	100 mA	1/20 sec	36″ SID	8 : 1 grid
	D.	65 kVp	200 mA	1/10 sec	36″ SID	no grid
22.	A.	70 kVp	500 mA	0.035 sec	40″ SID	6 : 1 grid
	B.	75 kVp	300 mA	0.025 sec	44″ SID	5 : 1 grid
	C.	80 kVp	100 mA	0.03 sec	36″ SID	8 : 1 grid
	D.	65 kVp	200 mA	0.02 sec	36″ SID	no grid
23.	A.	110 kVp	400 mA	0.10 sec	44″ SID	12 : 1 grid
	B.	120 kVp	600 mA	0.07 sec	40″ SID	16 : 1 grid
	C.	90 kVp	500 mA	0.15 sec	36″ SID	12 : 1 grid
	D.	100 kVp	800 mA	0.2 sec	40″ SID	16 : 1 grid
24.	A.	100 kVp	300 mA	0.15 sec	48″ SID	12 : 1 grid
	B.	120 kVp	200 mA	0.07 sec	44″ SID	16 : 1 grid
	C.	95 kVp	400 mA	0.2 sec	36″ SID	12 : 1 grid
	D.	100 kVp	400 mA	0.2 sec	30″ SID	16 : 1 grid

Determine the missing factor in the following radiographic techniques.

25.
200	mA		200	mA
0.05	sec		___	sec
80	kVp		92	kVp
12:1	grid		16:1	grid

26.
45	mAs		___	mAs
100	kVp		85	kVp
72-in	SID		60-in	SID
12:1	grid		8:1	grid

27.
200	mA		___	mA
100	msec		50	msec
70	kVp		80	kVp
no grid			8:1	grid

28.
30	mAs		___	mAs
78	kVp		90	kVp
40-in	SID		44-in	SID
6:1	grid		12:1	grid
400	screen speed		800	screen speed

29.
400	mA		300	mA
0.3	sec		___	sec
60	kVp		72	kVp
50	screen speed		100	screen speed
no grid			6:1	grid

30. An 8:1 grid is used with 85 kVp for 80 msec at 300 mA. What mAs would be required if you had to change to a 6:1 grid?

31. To determine the intensifying factor (IF) for a set of intensifying screens, divide the exposure used without screens by the exposure used with screens. If the exposure *with* screens requires 5 mAs and the exposure *without* screens requires 250 mAs, the intensification factor is _____.

32. When radiographing a 3-month-old child using a variable kVp technique, you should use 30% of the normal adult mAs. If the normal adult mAs for the examination requested is 60, the new mAs is _____.

33. To radiograph an extremity in a wet plaster cast requires 300% of the original mAs. If the technique called for 2 mAs for a radiograph of a hand and your patient had just been placed in a plaster cast that was still wet, you would have to use _____ mAs.

34. To radiograph an extremity in a dry plaster cast requires a 100% increase in the original mAs of 2. To radiograph the hand of a patient in a plaster cast that is 1 week old you would use _____ mAs.

35. Heat units for a single-phase x-ray machine are determined by multiplying kVp × mA × sec. The technique you are to use is 120 kVp at 400 mA for 0.035 sec. The heat units produced by this exposure are _____ .

36. One inch is equivalent to _____ meters.

37. Moving 180 cm in 1 hour is equivalent to moving _____ feet per second.

38. If 200 mA for 0.15 sec at a 40-in SID produces 4 R, an 80-in SID will produce _____ R.

39. To increase by 40% your original technique of 30 mAs requires a new mAs of _____ .

40. The technique chart calls for $\frac{1}{15}$ sec but your equipment requires decimal time settings. The decimal equivalent of $\frac{1}{15}$ is _____ .

41. A dose of 5 R per hour is equal to _____ R per minute and _____ R per second.

Fill in the conversion factors requested.

42. 10 Gy is equivalent to _____ rad.

43. 0.1 Sv is equivalent to _____ rem.

44. 10 rad is equivalent to _____ Gy.

45. 4 rem is equivalent to _____ Sv.

46. 36 in is equivalent to _____ cm.

47. 10 m is equivalent to _____ feet.

48. 30° C is equivalent to _____ ° F.

49. 98° F is equivalent to _____ ° C.

50. 48 lb is equivalent to _____ kg.

Determine the amount of geometric unsharpness (GU) in the following techniques:

51. FSS = 2.0
    OFD = 1.5 in
    FOD = 38.5 in
    GU = _____

52. FSS = 0.6
    FOD = 30 in
    SID = 36 in
    GU = _____

53. FSS = 3
    FOD = 70 in
    SID = 72 in
    GU = _____

54. FSS = 1
    OFD = 2 in
    FOD = 70 in
    GU = _____

55. Determine the size of the projected image of an object that measures 1 in if using an SID of 40 in and an FOD of 38 in.

56. Determine the projected image size of an object that measures 14 cm when using an SID of 108 cm and an FOD of 100 cm.

57. What will be the projected image size of a 2-in object if the OID is 0.5 in and the FOD is 60 in?

58. What will be the projected image size of a 4-in object if the OID is 1.5 in and the FOD is 38 in?

59. Determine the percentage of magnification if the OFD is 2 in and the FOD is 38 in.

60. Determine the percentage of magnification if the OFD is 4 in and the FOD is 72 in.

61. Determine the percentage of magnification if the OFD is 1 in and the FOD is 40 in.

62. Determine the magnification factor if the SID is 40 in and the FOD is 36 in.

63. Determine the magnification factor if the SID is 36 in and the FOD is 35 in.

64. Determine the percentage of magnification if the OFD is 1.5 in and the FOD is 35 in.

65. Determine the magnification factor if the SID is 72 in and the FOD is 68 in.

66. Convert 25 feet per second to meters per hour.

67. Convert 280 miles per hour to centimeters per second.

68. How many heat units would be produced on a single-phase radiographic unit using a technique of 90 kVp at 300 mA for 0.035 sec?

69. How many heat units would be produced on a three-phase (6-pulse) radiographic unit using a technique of 120 kVp at 600 mA for 0.005 sec?

70. How many heat units would be produced on a three-phase (12-pulse) radiographic unit using a technique of 120 kVp at 600 mA for 0.005 sec?

71. A series of six x-ray exposures is made on a single-phase unit with a technique of 75 kVp at 400 mA for 0.4 sec. What is the total number of heat units produced?

72. If a patient receives a radiation dose of 6 mR when radiographed at an SID of 40 in, what dose in mR would be received if an SID of 60 in were used?

73. If a patient receives a radiation dose of 2 mR when radiographed at an SID of 60 in, what dose in mR would be received if an SID of 40 in were used?

74. If a patient receives a radiation dose of 0.02 mR when radiographed at an SID of 36 in, what dose in mR would be received if an SID of 44 in were used?

75. If a patient receives a radiation dose of 0.5 mR when radiographed at an SID of 48 in, what dose in mR would be received if an SID of 40 in were used?

Using the graph below determine the missing factor for the exposures listed.

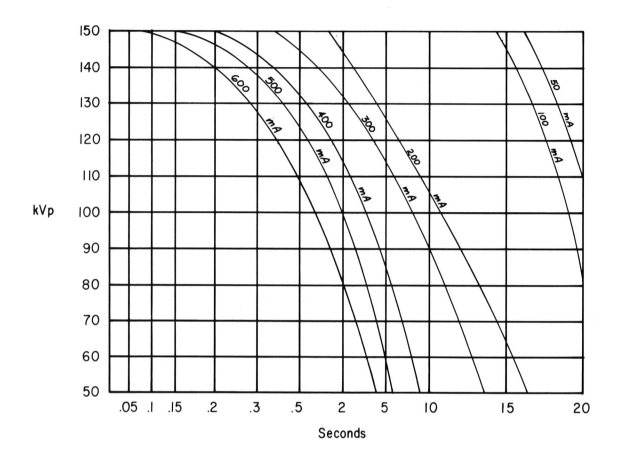

	kVp	mA	Maximum Exposure Time (sec)
76.	110	400	_____
77.	60	600	_____
78.	75	200	_____
79.	___	600	0.1
80.	100	___	2.0

81. If a circuit is connected in series with five elements of 1 ohm, 2 ohms, 3 ohms, 4 ohms, and 5 ohms, what is the total resistance?

82. Use the power rule to determine the watts produced by a voltage of 50 and a current of 100 amperes.

83. Use Ohm's law to determine the voltage of a circuit with 5 amperes flowing through a conductor with a resistance of 25 ohms.

84. If a circuit is connected in series with three elements of 2 ohms, 5 ohms, and 8 ohms, what is the total resistance?

85. Use the power rule to determine the watts produced by a voltage of 100 and a current of 50 amperes.

86. Use Ohm's law to determine the voltage of a circuit with 10 amperes flowing through a conductor with a resistance of 5 ohms.

87. What is the resistance of a circuit with a voltage of 10 and a current of 5 amperes?

88. Determine the amperes of a circuit with a potential difference of 5 volts and a resistance of 2 ohms.

89. A syringe must be prepared with contrast medium for a child who weighs 20 lb. The radiologist requests that the dose be prepared to deliver a concentration of 1 ml/kg body weight. How many cubic centimeters would you prepare for the injection?

90. The radiologist requests that a particular contrast agent be mixed with 250 ml of normal saline to create a 25% concentration. How much of the agent should be mixed with saline?

For the following problems determine the final kVp and mAs that should be used to achieve the requested results.

91. Original technique is 100 kVp at 600 mA for 0.07 sec. An 8:1 grid is used with a 40-in SID. Determine the technique needed to produce a radiograph that exhibits more contrast and twice the density.

92. Using the original factors in Problem 91, decrease the scale of contrast and cut the density 40%.

93. The original technique called for 75 kVp at 45 mAs. Without changing the density or scale of contrast, it is necessary to change from a 6:1 grid technique to an 8:1 grid and also to change the distance from 40 in to 30 in.

94. Using the original technique in Problem 93, decrease the contrast, use a 12:1 grid, and increase the density by 100%.

95. It is necessary to repeat the x-ray of a patient for whom you originally used 100 kVp at 200 mA for 0.02 sec, with a 12:1 grid at an SID of 44 in. You have to do this patient "portable" and must use an 8:1 grid at a 36-in distance.

96. The original technique calls for 90 kVp at 300 mA for 0.06 sec at a 40-in SID. Your radiograph needs a longer scale of contrast, twice the density, and you must use a 50-in SID. What time would be needed if you were required to use the 600-mA station? State both the decimal and fractional time.

97. The original technique calls for 90 kVp at 300 mA for 0.06 sec at a 40-in SID. Your radiograph needs a shorter scale of contrast, half the density, and you must use a 30-in SID. What time would be needed if you were required to use the 400-mA station? State both the decimal and fractional time.

98. The original technique calls for 90 kVp at 300 mA for 0.06 sec at a 40-in SID. Your radiograph needs more contrast, 50% less density, and you must use a 30-in SID. What time would be needed if you were required to use the 400-mA station? State both the decimal and fractional time.

99. The original technique calls for 75 kVp at 500 mA for 3/20 sec at a 40-in SID. Your radiograph needs less contrast, 50% more density, and you must use a 50-in SID. What time would be needed if you were required to use the 600-mA station? State both the decimal and fractional times.

100. The original technique calls for 110 kVp at 800 mA for 4/5 sec at a 72-in SID. Your radiograph needs more contrast, a 65% reduction in density, and you must use a 60-in SID. What time would be needed if you were required to use the 800-mA station? State both the decimal and fractional time.

ANSWERS TO SELECTED PROBLEMS

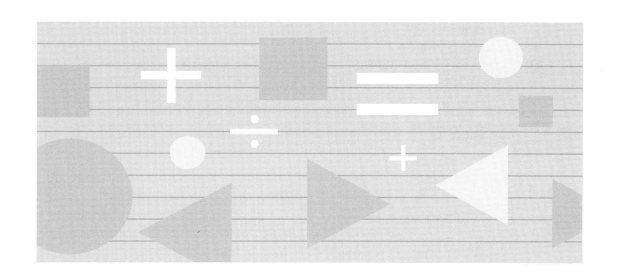

Section I Answers

▼ FRACTIONS ▼

1. $\frac{1}{8} \div \frac{4}{7} =$
   $\frac{1}{8} \times \frac{7}{4} = \frac{7}{32}$

2. $\frac{7}{9} = \frac{14}{18}$
   $-\frac{7}{18} = \frac{7}{18}$
   $\quad\quad = \frac{7}{18}$

3. $\frac{1}{4}$

4. $1\frac{3}{8} = 1\frac{1}{8} = \frac{33}{24}$
   $-\frac{2}{3} = \frac{2}{3} = \frac{16}{24}$
   $\quad\quad\quad = \frac{17}{24}$

5. $2\frac{3}{4} \div 2\frac{1}{9} =$
   $\frac{11}{4} \div \frac{19}{9} =$
   $\frac{11}{4} \times \frac{9}{19} = \frac{99}{76} = 1\frac{23}{76}$

6. $67\frac{1}{8} \times \frac{1}{4} =$
   $\frac{537}{8} \times \frac{1}{4} =$
   $\quad\quad \frac{537}{32} = 16\frac{25}{32}$

7. $\frac{5}{9}$

9. $30\frac{7}{12}$

11. $1\frac{29}{34}$

12. $\frac{6}{7} \times \frac{2}{9} \times \frac{14}{15} = \frac{8}{45}$

13. $\frac{7}{16} = \frac{7}{16}$
    $\frac{3}{4} = \frac{12}{16}$
    $\frac{1}{8} = \frac{2}{16}$
    $\quad = \frac{21}{16} = 1\frac{5}{16}$

15. $36\frac{1}{20}$

17. $55\frac{5}{12}$

19. $6\frac{5}{16}$

20. $(\frac{3}{7} + \frac{2}{5}) \times (\frac{7}{9} \div \frac{2}{3}) =$
    $\quad\quad \frac{29}{35} \times \frac{7}{6} = \frac{29}{30}$

21. $4^{5}/_{12}$

23. $7^{1}/_{30}$

25. $25^{23}/_{40}$

▼ DECIMALS ▼

1. $^8/_{10}$ = .8

3. 0.095

5. 0.03 = $^3/_{100}$

7. $^{41}/_{2000}$

9.   0.03
       3.2
     0.603
  +30.603
   34.508

11. 57.731

13. 1.689

14. 231.0000
    −0.9876
   230.0124

15. 12.5689

17.   1.634
    ×23
   4902
   3268
  37.582

19. 2.771

21. 16652.173

23. 7.712

25. 132.017

▼ PERCENTAGES ▼

1. $57\% = 0.57 = {}^{57}/_{100}$

2. $0.33 = {}^{33}/_{100}$

3. $1.2 = 1\frac{1}{5}$

4. $5.1 = 5\frac{1}{10}$

5.
```
   240        240
  ×0.3        +72
  ─────      ─────
  72.0        312
```

   or

```
   240
  ×1.3
  ─────
   720
   240
  ─────
   312.
```

7. 646

9. 300

11.
```
    360       360
  ×0.25       −90
  ─────      ─────
   1800       270
    720
  ─────
    90.
```

   or

```
    360
  ×0.75
  ─────
   1800
   2520
  ─────
    270.
```

13. 50

15. 59.5

17. $\begin{array}{r} 500 \\ \times 0.30 \\ \hline 150.00 \end{array}$

19. 262.5

21. 8

23. 450

▼ RATIOS AND PROPORTIONS ▼

1. $280 : 560 :: 1 : 2$
   $280 \times 2 = 560 \times 1$
   $560 = 560$

3. $3000 = 3000$

5. $21.78 = 21.78$

6. $x : 40 :: 10 : 400$
   $400x = 400$
   $x = 1$

7. $x = 45$

9. $x = \frac{1}{64}$

▼ ALGEBRA ▼

1. $a + b = cd$
   $a + b - b = cd - b$
   $a = cd - b$

3. $\dfrac{a}{b} = cd$

   $\dfrac{a}{b} \times b = cd \times b$

   $a = cdb$

5. $d = \dfrac{ab}{c}$

7. $a = \dfrac{cd}{b}$

9. $\dfrac{a}{b} = \dfrac{c}{d}$

   $bd \left(\dfrac{a}{b}\right) = bd \left(\dfrac{c}{d}\right)$

   $ad = bc$

   $\dfrac{ad}{c} = b$

11. $mA = \dfrac{mAs}{s}$

13. $x = 52$

15. $x = 18$

17. $x = 15$

19. $x = 36$

21. $x = {}^{7}/_{45}$

23. $-18 + 5x + 18 = 53 + 18$
   $5x = 71$
   $x = 14.2$

25. $x = 1$

▼ CIRCLES ▼

1. 3 in

3. 2 in

5. $c = 2\pi r$
$c = 2 \times 3.14 \times 3$
$c = 6.28 \times 3$
$c = 18.84$ in

6. $c = \pi d$
$c = 3.14 \times 1$
$c = 3.14$ m

7. $a = \pi r^2$
$a = 3.14 \times 2^2$
$a = 3.14 \times 4$
$a = 12.56$ cm^2

9. $a = \pi r^2$
$d = 1\ m$
$r = 0.5$ m
$a = 3.14 \times 5$
$a = 3.14 \times 0.25$
$a = 0.785$ m^2

11. $c = \pi d$
$d = \dfrac{c}{\pi}$
$d = \dfrac{31.4}{3.4}$
$d = 10$ in

12. $c = 2\pi r$
$r = \dfrac{c}{2}\pi$
$r = \dfrac{18.84}{2(3.14)}$
$r = \dfrac{18.84}{6.28}$
$r = 3$ cm

13. $c = 2\pi r$

$r = \dfrac{c}{2\pi}$

a. $r = \dfrac{9.42}{2(3.14)}$

$r = \dfrac{9.42}{6.28}$

$r = 1.5 \text{ ft}$

b. $a = 3.14(1.5)^2$
$a = 3.14(2.25)$
$a = 7.065 \text{ ft}^2$

15. $a = 254.34 \text{ in}^2$

▼ TRIANGLES ▼

1. $P = s_1 + s_2 + s_3$
   $P = 7 + 12 + 23$
   $P = 42$ cm

3. $P = s_1 + s_2 + s_3$
   60 in $= 15 + 15 + x$
   60 in $= 30 + x$
   30 in $= x$

5. $A = \frac{1}{2}bh$
   $A = \frac{1}{2} \times 10 \times 12$
   $A = 60$ cm^2

6. $A = 108$ in^2
   $A = \frac{3}{4}$ ft^2
   Remember that all terms must be converted to inches or feet; you cannot mix units in the same formula.

7. $A = 162$ in^2 or $1\frac{1}{8}$ ft^2

9. $c^2 = a^2 + b^2$
   $c^2 = (5\text{ in})^2 + (12\text{ in})^2$
   $c^2 = 25\text{ in}^2 + 144\text{ in}^2$
   $c^2 = 169$ in^2
   $c = 13$ in

10. $c^2 = a^2 + b^2$
    $c^2 = (6\text{ in})^2 + (8\text{ in})^2$
    $c^2 = 36\text{ in}^2 + 64\text{ in}^2$
    $c^2 = 100$ in^2
    $c = 10$ in

▼ RECTANGLES ▼

1. $P = 2L + 2W$
   $P = 2(9) + 2(4)$
   $P = 18 + 8$
   $P = 26$ in

2. $A = L \times W$
   $A = 3 \times 2$
   $A = 6$ ft^2

3. $\quad\quad\quad P = 2L + 2W$
   $46\ \text{in} = 2(16) + 2W$
   $46\ \text{in} = 32\ \text{in} + 2W$
   $46\ \text{in} - 32\ \text{in} = 2W$
   $14\ \text{in} = 2W$
   $7\ \text{in} = W$

5. $W = 7$ in

6. $\quad A = L \times W$
   $12 = L \times 3$
   $^{12}\!/_3 = L$
   $4\ \text{in} = L$

7. $P = 2L + 2W$
   $A = L \times W$

   To find L:

   $48 = 8 \times W$
   $6\ \text{in} = W$
   $P = 2(8) + 2(6)$
   $P = 16 + 12$
   $P = 28$ in

8. $\quad A = L \times W$
   $\quad\quad P = 2L + 2W$
   $42\ \text{in} = 2L + 2(6)$
   $42\ \text{in} = 2L + 12$
   $30\ \text{in} = 2L$
   $15\ \text{in} = L$
   $A = 15 \times 6$
   $A = 90$ in^2

9. $P = 120$ in

▼ SQUARES ▼

1. $P = 4 \times \text{side}$
   $P = 4 \times 1\frac{1}{2}$
   $P = 6 \text{ ft}$

2. $A = s^2$
   $s^2 = 169$
   $s = 13 \text{ in}$

3. $s = 3\frac{1}{2} \text{ ft}$

5. $A = s^2$
   $P = 4(\text{side})$
   $72 \text{ in} = 4s$
   $18 \text{ in} = s$

   To check:

   $A = (18 \text{ in})^2$
   $A = 324 \text{ in}^2$

▼ EXPONENTS ▼

1. $9 \times 9 = 81$

3. 5184

5. 1296

7. 2304

9. 64

11. 128

13. $6^3 = 6^{(7-4)} = 216$

14. $8^{(5-7)} = 8^{-2} = \frac{1}{8} \times \frac{1}{8} = \frac{1}{64}$

15. $2^{(4+6)} = 2^{-2} = \frac{1}{4}$

16. $3^{-1} = \frac{1}{3}$

17. $12^2 = 144$

19. 81

21. 72

23. 36

25. 44

27. 4^9

29. 8^7

▼ SCIENTIFIC NOTATION ▼

I.

    1. 2.5×10^1

    3. 3.608×10^3

    5. 7.83687×10^5

    7. 8.8×10^{-1}

    9. 8.07×10^{-2}

II.

    1. 18,000

    3. 7,800

    5. 8,700,000,000

    7. 0.00000089

    9. 0.00385

▼ MEASUREMENTS ▼

1. 38.1 cm

3. 182.88 cm

5. 32 oz

7. 107.6° F

9. 160,934.4

11. 0.04 sec

13. 0.005 sec

15. 35 msec

17. 300 msec

19. 600 msec

Section II Answers

▼ mAs CONVERSIONS ▼

A.

    1. mAs = mA × s(time)
       $400 \times \frac{1}{120} = 3.33 = 3\frac{1}{3}$

    3. 100

    5. $1.25 = 1\frac{1}{4}$

    6. $6.66 = 6\frac{2}{3}$

    7. 30

    9. 240

   10. $12.5 = 12\frac{1}{2}$

B.

    1. $10.5 = 10\frac{1}{2}$

    3. 6

    5. 1

    7. 21

    9. $1.75 = 1\frac{3}{4}$

C.

    1. $mA = \dfrac{mAs}{s}$

       $mA = \dfrac{6.66}{0.067}$

      $mA = 99.40$
      $mA = 100$

    3. 500

    5. 400

7. 500

9. 300

D.

1. $T = \dfrac{mAs}{mA}$

   $T = \dfrac{1.25}{100} = \dfrac{1}{80} = 0.0125$

3. $\frac{1}{50} = 0.02$

5. $\frac{1}{100} = 0.01$

7. $\frac{1}{80} = 0.0125$

9. $\frac{2}{5} = 0.4$

▼ INVERSE SQUARE LAW ▼

I. $\dfrac{\text{New mAs}}{\text{Old mAs}} = \dfrac{\text{New distance } (D_2{}^2)}{\text{Old distance } (D_1{}^2)}$

1. $\dfrac{x}{400} = \dfrac{60 \text{ in}^2}{40 \text{ in}^2}$

$\dfrac{x}{400} = \dfrac{3600}{1600}$

$16x = 14400$

$x = 900$

3. 104.166

5. 50.625

7. 403.33

9. 8.698

II.

Step 1:

Step 2:

1. 100 mA at $\dfrac{1}{2} = 50$ mAs $\dfrac{\text{mAs}}{\text{mA}} = \text{s}$

$\dfrac{x}{50} = \dfrac{44 \text{ in}^2}{40 \text{ in}^2}$ $\text{mA} = \text{s}$

$\dfrac{x}{50} = \dfrac{1536}{1600}$

$1600x = 96800$ $200 = {}^3\!/_{10}$

$x = 60.5$ $300 = {}^1\!/_5$ } Examples of possible answers

$400 = {}^3\!/_{20}$

$600 = {}^1\!/_{10}$

2. 12.5 mAs   8.68 mAs   50 mA = ⅙ = 8.33 mAs

or

300 mA = $^1\!/_{30}$ = 10 mAs

3. 21 mAs   39.05 mAs   600 mA = $^1\!/_{15}$

5. 16.66 mAs   11.59 mAs   1000 mA = $^1\!/_{80}$

III.

1.	45 mAs	31.25 mAs	300 mA at 0.1 sec
3.	200 mAs	162 mAs	800 mA at 0.2 sec
5.	18.75 mAs	50.2 mAs	100 mA at 0.5 sec

IV.

1. $\dfrac{\text{New intensity}}{\text{Old intensity}} = \dfrac{\text{Old distance}^2\ (D_1{}^2)}{\text{New distance}^2\ (D_2{}^2)}$

$\dfrac{x}{5\text{ mR}} = \dfrac{40\text{ in}^2}{36\text{ in}^2}$

$\dfrac{x}{5} = \dfrac{1600}{1296}$

$1296x = 8000$

$x = 6.172\text{ mR}$

3. 3.55 mR

5. 23.24 mR

7. 8.47 mR

9. 2.77 mR

▼ DENSITY ▼

1.
```
   60 mAs              60        60 mAs
  ×0.6        or     ×0.4        −24
  36.0 mAs           24.0        36 mAs
```

2. 300 mA at ⅕ = 60 mAs (Original mAs)
   60 mAs × 75% = 45 mAs (New mAs)

3. 22.5 mAs

4. 7.5 mAs

   * Note: A 100% increase would equal 5 mAs; therefore a 200% increase would require 10 mAs.

5. 19.5 mAs

6. 500 mA at 0.05 = 25 mAs

```
     25
    ×0.7
    17.5 mAs
```

$$s = \frac{mAs}{mA}$$

$$s = \frac{17.5}{500}$$

$$s = 0.035$$

7. 0.3 or ³⁄₁₀

   * Note: Because 192 mAs is not achievable, 180 mAs is the closest possible mAs to 192.

▼ CONTRAST ▼

I.

1. 60 kVp × 115% = 69 kVp
   300 mA × ³⁄₂ s = 45 mAs
   45 mAs × ½ = 22.5 mAs

3. sec = 0.05
   kVp = 115

5. mA = 24.9 or 25
   kVp = 109.25

II.

1. 120 kVp × 85% = 102 kVp
   200 mA × ¹⁄₁₅ s = 13.33 mAs
   13.33 × 2 = 26.66 mAs

3. sec = 0.6
   kVp = 93.5

5. mA = 999.6 or 1000
   kVp = 97.75 or 98

III.

1. 100 kVp × 85% = 85 kVp
   600 mA for 0.035 sec = 21 mAs

   600 mA for 0.035 sec could still be used, since reducing 100 kVp by 15% is equivalent to cutting the density in half.

3. 80.5 kVp
   2 mAs
   200 mA
   0.01 sec

▼ SCREEN CONVERSION ▼

1. 100-speed system to 400 rare earth = ¼ mAs
   80 mAs × ¼ = 20 mAs

3. 280 mAs

5. 15 mAs

7. 6 mAs

9. 150 mAs

▼ GRID RATIOS ▼

1. Grid ratio $= \dfrac{h}{w}$

   Grid ratio $= \dfrac{1.2}{0.1} = 12$

   Grid ratio $= 12 : 1$

3. $5 : 1$

5. $10 : 1$

▼ GRID CONVERSION ▼

1. $mAs_2 = mAs_1 \left(\dfrac{G_2}{G_1}\right)$

    $x = 30(5/4)$
    $x = 37.5$

3. 60 mAs

5. 25 mAs

7. 100 mAs

9. 140 mAs

▼ GEOMETRIC UNSHARPNESS ▼

1. Geometric unsharpness $= \dfrac{\text{FSS} \times \text{OFD}}{\text{FOD}}$

$x = \dfrac{1.5 \times 3}{32}$

$x = \dfrac{4.5}{32}$

$x = 0.14$ in

3. FFD − OFD = FOD
   44 − 2 = 42 (FOD)

$x = \dfrac{2 \times 2}{42}$

$x = \dfrac{4}{42}$

$x = 0.095$

4. FFD − FOD = OFD
   48 − 38 = 10 (OFD)

$x = \dfrac{1 \times 10}{38}$

$x = \dfrac{10}{38}$

$x = 0.26$

5. 0.21

7. 0.75

9. 0.03

11. A

13. A

15. B

17. C

▼ MAGNIFICATION UNSHARPNESS ▼

1. $\dfrac{OS}{IS} = \dfrac{FOD}{FFD}$

   $\dfrac{7 \text{ in}}{x} = \dfrac{40 \text{ in}}{44 \text{ in}}$

   $40x = 308$
   $x = 7.7 \text{ in}$

3. 14.1 in

5. $MF = \dfrac{FFD}{FOD}$

   $^{40}\!/_{36} = 1.1$

7. 1.1

8. $\dfrac{OFD}{FOD} \times 100$

   $^{3}\!/_{41} \times 100$
   $^{300}\!/_{41} = 7.3\%$

   or

   $^{3}\!/_{41} = 0.0731$
   $0.0731 \times 100 = 7.3\%$

9. 20%

11. Step 1: $\dfrac{OFD}{FOD} \times 100 = \%$ magnification

    $^{2}\!/_{38} \times 100 = 5.26\%$

    Step 2: Object size + % magnification = IS
    $10 + (10 \times 5.26\%) =$
    $10 + 0.526 = 10.526 \text{ in}$

13. 16.4 in

15. 2.54 cm = 1 in
    $26.73 \div 2.54 = 10.5 \text{ in}$

16. Step 1: FFD − OFD = FOD
    $72 - 2 = 70 \text{ in}$

    Step 2: $\dfrac{OFD}{FOD} \times 100 = \%$ magnification

    $^{2}\!/_{70} \times 100 = 2.9\%$

17. Step 1: FFD − FOD = OFD
$\qquad$ 60 − 56 = 4 in (OFD)

Step 2: $\dfrac{OFD}{FOD} \times 100 = \%$ magnification

$\qquad$ $\frac{4}{56} \times 100 = 7.14\%$ magnification

Step 3: 0.5 + % magnification = IS
$\qquad$ 15 + 7.14% = 16.1 in

19. 1.02

▼ SYSTÈME INTERNATIONAL ▼

I.

1. 2 Gy
   $200 \times 0.01 = 2$ Gy

3. 0.0005 Sv

5. 12.9×10^{-4}

II.

1. 1.1000 rem
   $10 \div 0.01 = 1000$ rem

3. 50,000 rad

5. 2.7×10^{10} Ci

Section III Answers

▼ PRACTICAL APPLICATIONS ▼

1. 0.02 sec

3. 20 mAs

5. 600 mA at 0.08 sec

7. 0.07 sec

9. 0.1 sec (40 mAs)

11. 0.03 sec (24 mAs)

13. 0.067 sec (40 mAs)

15. 0.035 sec or $\frac{1}{20}$ sec (3.35 mAs)

17. 5 mAs

19. 10 mAs

21. D

23. D

25. 0.03 sec

27. 800 mA

29. 120 mAs

31. 50 IF

33. 6 mAs

35. 1,680 HU

37. 0.0016 ft/sec

39. 42 mAs

41. 0.08 R/min and 0.001 R/sec

43. 10 rem

45. 0.04 Sv

47. 32.8 ft

49. 36.66° C

51. 0.077

53. 0.085

55. 1.05 in

57. 2.016 in

59. 5.26%

61. 2.5%

63. 1.028

65. 5.88%

67. 125,171.2 cm/sec

69. 486 HU

71. 72,000 HU

73. 4.5 mR

75. 0.72 mR

77. 3 sec

79. 148 kVp

81. 15 ohms

83. 125 volts

85. 5,000 watts

87. 2 ohms

89. 44 cc

91. 85 kVp at 168 mAs

93. 75 kVp at 33.75 mAs

95. 2.14 mAs

97. 0.25 sec or 1/40 sec

99. 0.15 sec or 3/20 sec

A P P E N D I X B

mAs
TABLE

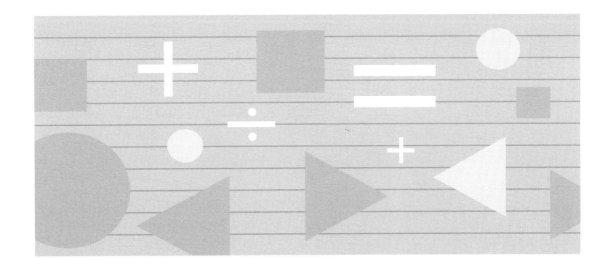

Time Decimals	Time Fractions	0.25	50	100	200
0.0083	1/120	0.21	0.42	0.83	1.66
0.007	—	0.18	0.35	0.7	1.4
0.01	1/100	0.25	0.5	1.	2.
0.0125	1/80	0.31	0.63	1.25	2.5
0.0167	1/60	0.42	0.84	1.67	3.34
0.02	1/50	0.5	1.	2.	4.
0.025	1/40	0.63	1.25	2.5	5.
0.033	1/30	0.83	1.65	3.3	6.6
0.035	—	0.88	1.75	3.5	7.
0.05	1/20	1.25	2.5	5.	10.
0.067	1/15	1.68	3.35	6.7	13.4
0.07	—	1.75	3.5	7.	14.
0.083	1/12	2.08	4.15	8.3	16.6
0.1	1/10	2.5	5.	10.	20.
0.125	1/8	3.13	6.25	12.5	25.
0.133	2/15	3.33	6.65	13.3	26.6
0.15	3/20	3.75	7.5	15.	30.
0.167	1/6	4.18	8.35	16.7	33.4
0.2	1/5	5.	10.	20.	40.
0.25	1/4	6.25	12.5	25.	50.
0.3	3/10	7.5	15.	30.	60.
0.35	—	8.75	17.5	35.	70.
0.4	2/5	10.	20.	40.	80.
0.5	1/2	12.5	25.	50.	100.
0.7	—	17.5	35.	70.	140.
0.75	3/4	18.75	37.5	75.	150.
0.8	4/5	20.	40.	80.	160.
0.9	9/10	22.5	45.	90.	180.
1.0	1	25.	50.	100.	200.
1.5	1½	37.5	75.	150.	300.
2.0	2	50.	100.	200.	400.

Milliamperes

300	400	500	600	800	1000
2.5	3.32	4.15	5.	6.64	8.3
2.1	2.8	3.5	4.2	5.6	7.0
3.	4.	5.	6.	8.	10.0
3.75	5.	6.25	7.5	10.	12.5
5.	6.68	8.35	10.	13.36	16.7
6.	8.	10.	12.	16.	20.
7.5	10.	12.5	15.	20.	25.
10.	13.2	16.5	20.	26.4	33.
10.5	14.	17.5	21.	28.	35.
15.	20.	25.	30.	40.	50.
20.1	26.8	33.5	40.2	53.6	67.
21.	28.	35.	42.	56.	70.
25.	33.2	41.5	50.	66.4	83.
30.	40.	50.	60.	80.	100.
37.5	50.	62.5	75.	100.	125.
40.	53.2	66.5	80.	106.4	133.
45.	60.	75.	90.	120.	150.
50.	66.8	83.5	100.	133.6	167.
60.	80.	100.	120.	160.	200.
75.	100.	125.	150.	200.	250.
90.	120.	150.	180.	240.	300.
105.	140.	175.	210.	280.	350.
120.	160.	200.	240.	320.	400.
150.	200.	250.	300.	400.	500.
210.	280.	350.	420.	560.	700.
225.	300.	375.	450.	600.	750.
240.	320.	400.	480.	640.	800.
270.	360.	450.	540.	720.	900.
300.	400.	500.	600.	800.	1000.
450.	600.	750.	900.	1200.	1500.
600.	800.	1000.	1200.	1600.	2000.

INDEX

Note: Page numbers in *italics* refer to illustrations.